RESEARCH IN COMMUNICATION SCIENCES AND DISORDERS: METHODS FOR SYSTEMATIC INQUIRY

RESEARCH IN COMMUNICATION SCIENCES AND DISORDERS: METHODS FOR SYSTEMATIC INQUIRY

Lauren K. Nelson

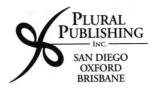

PLURAL
PUBLISHING
INC.

SAN DIEGO
OXFORD
BRISBANE

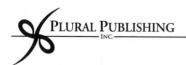

5521 Ruffin Road
San Diego, CA 92123

e-mail: info@pluralpublishing.com
Web site: http://www.pluralpublishing.com

49 Bath Street
Abingdon, Oxfordshire OX14 1EA
United Kingdom

Typeset in 10½/13 Garamond by Flanagan's Publishing Services, Inc.
Printed in the United States of America by McNaughton & Gunn, Inc.

For permission to use material from this text, contact us by
Telephone: (866) 758-7251
Fax: (888) 758-7255
e-mail: permissions@pluralpublishing.com

Every attempt has been made to contact the copyright holders for material originally printed in another source. If any have been inadvertently overlooked, the publishers will gladly make the necessary arrangements at the first opportunity.

Library of Congress Cataloging-in-Publication Data:
Nelson, Lauren.
  Research in communication sciences and disorders : methods for systematic inquiry / Lauren Nelson.
     p. ; cm.
  Includes bibliographical references and index.
  ISBN-13: 978-1-59756-246-1 (alk. paper)
  ISBN-10: 1-59756-246-7 (alk. paper)
  1. Communicative disorders–Research–Methodology. 2. Audiology–Research–Methodology. 3. Communication–Research–Methodology. I. Title.
  [DNLM: 1. Communication Disorders. 2. Biomedical Research–methods. 3. Research Design. WL 340.2 N427r 2008]
  RC423.N353 2008
  362.196'8550072–dc22
                          2008025803

Contents

Preface

Teaching a research course for graduate students in communication sciences and disorders has been my privilege for several years. Only a small number of these students planned to pursue a career in research and/or higher education, and the majority anticipated working in a clinical setting as an audiologist or speech-language pathologist. At the beginning of the course I have given students an opportunity to express concerns about the topics they expected to cover. Over the years the students reported very similar concerns. Many worried that they would have difficulty understanding the content of research articles, particularly the statistical information. Others described prior frustration with their attempts to read research reports because they spent considerable time rereading material that was difficult to understand. Many students were uneasy about finding a "good" topic for their own graduate research project. A few even admitted that motivation was a concern because they expected the topics to be less than exciting.

The students and I tackled these concerns in several ways. Recognizing that the way of thinking that underlies scientific inquiry was highly similar to the way audiologists and speech-language pathologists think about assessment and treatment of persons with communication disorders was an important first step. The students found their motivation by understanding that high quality research stems from genuine curiosity and interest about a topic, and by recog-

nizing the importance of strong evidence in providing clinical services. They discovered that research was essential for high quality clinical practice, that research in the field of communication sciences and disorders took many forms, and that audiologists and speech-language pathologists needed skills to investigate the existing research base to find good evidence to support their clinical decisions.

The concerns my students expressed about research and the strategies we developed to address those concerns were the basis for this text. The knowledge and skills one needs to engage in empirical research and to use research in clinical practice are comparable, and that is how these topics are presented in this text. Rather than treating empirical research and searching for clinical evidence as separate topics, this text presents both as different applications of a process of scientific inquiry. The order of the chapters reflects the steps a researcher or clinician might complete when conducting a scientific investigation. Chapter 1 introduces the topic of scientific inquiry and its different applications in the field of communication sciences and disorders. Because ethical practice is a primary concern for both clinicians and researchers, Chapter 2 covers ethical issues that affect the design, conduct, and utilization of research. Chapter 3 describes how researchers and clinicians might formulate questions as the starting point for their investigations. Some of these questions might be answered in the existing literature and others might be refined based on the existing literature. Thus, Chapter 4 addresses the information you might need to conduct a good quality literature search. Chapter 5 and Chapter 6 cover the different types of research that are common in the field of communication sciences and disorders and the relationship between these types of research and the evidence audiologists and speech-language pathologists need to support their clinical endeavors. Chapter 7 discusses how researchers select persons to participate in research and issues associated with that process. Chapter 8 and Chapter 9 describe the analysis of research data using various statistical procedures. The final chapter, Chapter 10, describes how researchers and clinicians use the information gathered through their investigations. For researchers this often involves preparation of a research report to disseminate to other professionals, and for clinicians it usually leads to a decision about the most appropriate assessment and treatment approaches for their clients.

Each chapter includes examples from the field of communication sciences and disorders to illustrate important concepts. Review questions are included at the end of each chapter along with some suggestions for additional learning activities. Where appropriate, the learning activities include a list of research articles from journals in communication sciences and disorders that illustrate topics covered in the chapter. The learning activities could serve as homework assignments or in some cases as the focus of in-class discussions. In my own courses, we use the review questions in small group activities. I particularly enjoy observing students explain difficult questions to each other and doing so in a way that illustrates their own mastery of the concepts.

CHAPTER 1

Empirical and Nonempirical Research: An Overview

For many students, learning that they need to complete a research course is a cause of considerable anxiety. Perhaps you are someone who views research as a requirement to endure rather than as a topic to embrace; or perhaps you acknowledge the importance of research in communication sciences and disorders but consider it something that others with unique talents undertake. One aim of this introductory chapter is to establish the fact that research encompasses many different kinds of activities, some of which you already engage in. Further, the knowledge and skills we need to be effective researchers are not necessarily unique talents but often parallel the processes and procedures employed by audiologists and speech-language pathologists.

Systematic Inquiry

One way to view research is as a process of *systematic inquiry*. Making an inquiry involves asking a question and then engaging in a process to determine the answer to that question. Asking and answering questions is at the heart of research endeavors. Research is systematic because the approach

you use to find answers has predetermined procedures, and these procedures are carried out in a regular, orderly manner.

One approach to systematic inquiry is the *scientific method*. This method involves a series of steps that lead from identifying a problem and formulating a question to discovering possible answers to that question. Peterson and Marquardt (1994, p. 26) identified the following six steps in this process:

1. Definition of the problem
2. Development of hypotheses to be tested
3. Development of a procedure for testing the hypotheses
4. Collection of data
5. Analysis of data
6. Support or rejection of hypotheses

You would expect to find the steps of the scientific method in a research text. However, Peterson and Marquardt included these steps in their appraisal and diagnosis text (*Appraisal and Diagnosis of Speech and Language Disorders*). These authors observed that diagnosis involves a way of thinking that parallels the method scientists employ in their experimental research. When faced with a clinical problem, such as a person referred for an evaluation, audiologists and speech-language pathologists gather and analyze data to test a hypothesis. In the case of a speech, language, or hearing evaluation, the hypotheses relate to whether or not someone has a disorder, and the nature of that disorder. Although the types of questions or hypotheses differ, both clinical practice and research involve ways of thinking and problem-solving that are systematic in nature. When the process of inquiry is systematic, both clinicians and scientists have greater confidence that the information they provide is accurate and trustworthy, whether providing that information to individual clients and their families or to the scientific community.

Some Roles for Research

Scientific research has many roles in the fields of audiology and speech-language pathology. Perhaps the most basic role is to satisfy scientific curiosity. Researchers in communication sciences and disorders regularly participate in a process of identifying unanswered questions and designing information gathering procedures to answer those questions. Researchers focus on questions they regard as important for understanding the nature of human communication, the underlying physiology of speaking and hearing, the causes of speech, language, and hearing disorders, and so forth. Researchers who are motivated primarily by scientific curiosity might still include persons with speech, language, or hearing disorders in their studies and conduct research that has implications for assessing and treating communication disorders. For example, one way researchers learned about the neurological bases of speech and language was by including persons with aphasia in their studies. These types of studies provided information about the effects of brain lesions on

speech and language use but did not necessarily lead directly to specific assessment or treatment recommendations.

Research is also valuable in guiding clinical practice in audiology and speech-language pathology. Sometimes audiologists and speech-language pathologists are motivated to conduct research because of unanswered questions they encounter in their clinical practice. Silverman (1998) used the term *clinician-investigator* to refer to audiologists and speech-language pathologists whose primary responsibility is providing clinical services but who also engage in research in their profession. In many ways such individuals are ideally positioned to conduct research that guides the way audiologists speech-language pathologists diagnose and treat communication disorders. Clinician-investigators have firsthand knowledge regarding information that is lacking and also work with clients in their professional practice who would be most representative of children and adults with speech, language, and hearing disorders.

The notion of using research to guide clinical practice is important even for audiologists and speech-language pathologists who do not conduct their own original research. In recent years a strong movement toward use of scientific evidence to make decisions emerged in both the fields of medicine and education. Because audiologists and speech-language pathologists are employed in medical and educational settings, this movement has encompassed those fields as well. The term *evidence-based practice* refers to an approach in which clinicians use the best available scientific evidence to guide their decisions about how to evaluate and treat persons with communication disorders. According to Sacket, Rosenberg, Gray, Haynes, and Richardson (1996, p. 71 as cited in ASHA, 2004, p. 1), when clinicians engage in evidence-based practice, they are making client decisions by

" . . . integrating individual clinical expertise with the best available external evidence from systematic research."[1]

When audiologists and speech-language pathologists participate in evidence-based practice, they might do so by consulting an existing evidence review. Such reviews usually are prepared by a panel of experts. They are published in professional journals or perhaps published in electronic format on a Web site. Some examples include a review of rehabilitation for acquired brain injury (Turner-Stokes, Disler, Nair, & Wade, 2005), treatment for aphasia (Robey, 1998), the cost-effectiveness of digital hearing aids (Taylor, Paisley, & Davis, 2001), and intervention for language delays (Law, Garrett, & Nye, 2004). Many examples of evidence reviews published from 1997 through 2006 are documented by the American Speech-Language-Hearing Association (ASHA, 2007). Sometimes audiologists and speech-language pathologists conduct individual evidence searches on behalf of a particular client. Such searches begin with a client-specific question and culminate with review, evaluation, and application of existing research. Clinicians might use existing research literature when answering questions such as which of two treatment approaches produced the most improvement in the shortest time, whether a particular diagnostic procedure yields results that are accurate and reliable, or what is the most effective treatment for a client with a specific diagnosis. Evidence-based practice reflects a movement away from sole reliance on expert opinion toward an approach that relies on careful consideration of research evidence in conjunction with clinical expertise and client/family considerations (Gallagher, 2002).

Another reason audiologists and speech-language pathologists engage in research is for program evaluation and support. This type of research is conducted at a local level sometimes in response to external requirements and sometimes due to local initiatives. For example, a medical center might evaluate the quality of its programs and services by comparing them to a set of nationally recognized standards. Professionals employed in educational settings are very much aware of the use of student achievement testing to evaluate school programs. Again, such evaluation involves comparisons to state and national standards purported to reflect the quality of school programs. At other times program evaluation questions emerge from local rather than state or national initiatives. For example, a medical center might conduct consumer satisfaction research with the goal of improving its programs and services and increasing the likelihood that consumers choose that medical center as their health care provider. A school district might conduct program evaluation research after making changes to curriculum or teaching practices to determine if these changes led to improvements in student learning and achievement. Although professionals, such as audiologists, speech-language pathologists, nurses, physicians, and teachers, often debate the best approaches for program evaluation, nearly all agree that research of this type plays an important role in their professions.

Scientific research also may influence public policy, particularly policy regarding the allocation of resources. When research evidence is particularly strong, legislators and policy makers may consider this evidence in making decisions about spending public funds. An example of this is the

---

[1]The American Speech-Language Hearing Association (2005) position statement on evidence based practice can be found in the document, *Evidence-Based Practice in Communication Disorders* [Position Statement], available from http://www.asha.org. In this document ASHA established the position that audiologists and speech-language pathologists should engage in evidence based practice to assure provision of the highest quality clinical services.

growth of publicly funded early childhood education for all 3- and 4-year-olds. One reason for the increase in public funding is research that consistently demonstrated that children who attended good quality preschool programs performed better in school and were more successful in their later lives. The research actually demonstrated that the funds spent early in childhood were offset by savings that occurred later through reduced educational spending on special services and reduced need for public assistance in adulthood.

Research that demonstrates how a service or program impacts society is sometimes referred to as cost-effectiveness or cost-benefit research. Cost-effectiveness research looks at the cost of a program or service relative to the outcomes produced (Barnett, 2000). For example, if different treatment programs or different technology varied in cost, an audiologist or speech-language pathologist would probably want to know that the more expensive approach produced better outcomes for their clients. Cost-benefit research looks at the cost of a program or service relative to its impact on costs that occur later in life. For preschool education, the analysis included documentation of the cost of the educational program and long-term follow-up of the children who participated. The long-term follow-up revealed actual cost benefits to society in several different ways. For example, children who received early childhood education were less likely to need special education services during the school years, were less likely to need other public services such as juvenile detention, were less likely to participate in public assistance programs as adults, and typically earned more income per year as adults (Barnett, 2000). Thus, individuals who advocated for public funding of early childhood education could point to a body of research that suggested such programs produced a net financial benefit to society that greatly offset the initial cost. Audiologists and speech-language pathologists would profit from a body of research demonstrating the benefits of our programs.

Types of Research

Taking some time to peruse published research in audiology and speech-language pathology, such as that found in our professional journals, would reveal many forms of research. Generally research studies share at least one similarity—a question that needs an answer or problem that needs a solution. However, how researchers formulate their questions or how they plan and conduct their studies can be quite different. In this section we will consider some of the terminology researchers use to characterize these differences.

Most of the time when professionals in the fields of audiology and speech-language pathology use the term *research*, they are referring to *empirical* research. Empirical research involves the collection of new information or data through observation and measurement of behavior and/or physical properties (Trochim & Donnelly, 2007). Review of recent issues of professional journals in communication sciences and disorders revealed several ways that human behavior was observed and measured, such as speech samples (Sawyer & Yairi, 2006), survey responses (MacNeil, Lui, Stone, & Farrell, 2007; Skahan, Watson, & Lof, 2007), listener ratings (Spielman, Ramig, Mahler, Halpern, & Gavin, 2007), and test scores (van Kleeck, Vander Woude, & Hammett, 2006), as well as several ways of measuring physical properties, such as speaker sound pressure levels (Spielman et al., 2007), tongue strength and endurance (Stierwalt & Youmans, 2007), and electromyographic waveform displays (Yiu, Verdolini, & Chow, 2005). Examples of research that is nonempirical might include a carefully constructed theoretical analysis or a systematic review of a body of research.

Another way to characterize different forms of research is the distinction between *qualitative* and *quantitative* research. Qualitative research and quantitative research differ with regard to the way questions or problems are formulated and investigated. However, a commonly identified difference is in the type of information or data a researcher gathers. In qualitative research data often includes verbal information. This might take the form of highly detailed descriptions of a person's behavior or perhaps direct quotes of a person's statements. Quantitative research, as you might expect, relates to numerical information such as frequency counts and measures of size or other physical properties. Sometimes researchers gather both types of data and report both numerical and verbal information.

Within the category of quantitative research we often make a distinction between studies that are *experimental* and those that are *nonexperimental*. In experimental research, researchers identify one or more factors that they will manipulate or control during the experiment. For example, a researcher might be comparing different approaches for improving a person's communication abilities and could manipulate how much or what type of approach participants experience. The researcher manipulates or controls the conditions so that some participants have a different experience during the experiment than others. According to Patten (2007), a *true experiment* meets two criteria. The first is the researcher's creation of different conditions or experiences by manipulating one or more factors during the experiment, and the second is that the conditions participants experience are determined randomly. A true experiment has

random assignment of the participants to different experimental groups. Experimental research that lacks random assignment to groups is sometimes referred to as *quasi-experimental* research. Generally speaking, a study that meets both standards, experimental manipulation and random assignment, provides stronger evidence than a quasi-experimental study.

One of the most common kinds of experiments is one in which a researcher compares the performance of two groups, each experiencing a different experimental manipulation or treatment. In audiology and speech-language pathology such comparison might involve traditional treatment as compared to some new treatment approach. As noted, when the participants are divided at random into groups, the study is considered a true experiment. However, sometimes researchers find it impractical or impossible to assign their participants randomly. Perhaps the researchers want to compare two different classroom-based interventions. Children in school settings are seldom assigned to their classrooms in a random manner. Therefore, if researchers decide to conduct the experiment with two existing classrooms, they are conducting quasi-experimental research rather than a true experiment.

In contrast with experimental research, nonexperimental research includes a wide variety of studies in which the researcher investigates existing conditions. Some forms of nonexperimental research are descriptive in nature. Studies that provide information about the typical communication behaviors of persons of various ages fall into this category. Such studies might include measures based on speech and language samples, measures of physical properties of speech such as fundamental frequency or intensity, as well as psychoacoustic responses to speech. Some examples of nonexperimental research include case studies, surveys, studies of relationships or correlations between measures, as well as comparison studies (Patten, 2007). In comparison studies researchers include groups of persons with preexisting differences, rather than create differences via an experimental manipulation. Some examples include comparisons of 3-year-olds and 5-year-olds, persons with a particular type of hearing loss and persons with normal hearing, adults with functional voice disorders and those with normal voices, or children with specific language impairment and those with typical language.

Another important distinction for research in communication sciences and disorders is the difference between *group* and *single subject* research. This difference is not associated with the number of research participants in a literal way. That is, one might encounter a small group study with just five participants in each group, or one might encounter single subject research with several participants. Nor is single subject research the equivalent of a case study. Case studies involve nonexperimental, descriptive research, whereas single subject research is experimental in nature. The most important differences between group and single subject research concern how participants are treated during the study and how their data are reported. In single subject research, a participant experiences both the experimental and control conditions, and results for each participant are reported separately. When experimental and control conditions are compared in group research, usually the participants in one group experience the experimental condition and the participants in another group experience the control condition. The results from group research are aggregated and reported for each of the comparison groups and not for individual participants.

Variables

Two additional terms will be useful for understanding how researchers talk about their studies. Usually researchers have identified some characteristic or manipulation they want to investigate. The characteristic or manipulation the researcher wants to study is called the *independent variable*. In experimental research the independent variable might be an experience such as receiving a treatment or a way of presenting information that the researcher manipulates. In nonexperimental research the independent variable might be an existing characteristic such as the presence or absence of a communication disorder or the age of the participants. Often the independent variable has two or more categories or levels that the researcher wants to compare in some way (Patten, 2007). Keep in mind that experimental and nonexperimental studies may have more than one independent variable, and sometimes researchers study the effects of both an experimental manipulation and an existing characteristic in the same investigation. An example of this would be a researcher who studies the effects of a treatment manipulation, such as giving feedback in two different ways, for children in two different age groups. The researcher could determine in a random way which participants receive a particular type of feedback during their treatment, but the age of the children is an existing characteristic that cannot be manipulated.

When researchers want to compare the performance of their participants, they need to identify ways of measuring that performance. The measures that researchers use to determine the outcomes of their experimental or nonexperimental research are called *dependent variables*. In a sense, you might think of independent variables as the inputs and dependent variables as the outputs of the research. If the experimental manipulation or existing characteristics made a difference, researchers will see these differences in the values of their dependent variables or outcome measures.

Getting Started with Research

One of the best ways to become familiar with the various types of research is to read the research reports published in our professional journals. Sometimes students express frustration with the notion of reading professional research. They find the articles highly detailed and confusing. When reading a research report, keep in mind that the key information in nearly any such report is a question or problem the researcher investigated and the answer(s) provided by the researcher's observations or data. Thus, the most important goal in reading a research report is to find out the research question(s) and to learn what the author(s) wrote in answering those questions.

Silverman (1998) suggested a five-part strategy for reading and taking notes on a research article. He suggested you needed to obtain complete reference information, the research question(s), a brief description of the procedures, a brief description of the outcome measures or observations, and the answer to the research question. Some examples of this question and answer format are included on pages 7–9 in Silverman's book.

One approach you might consider is to read the article in a nonlinear way. Most research reports follow a very similar structure. The articles include an introduction and review of literature, methods, results, discussion, and summary sections. Most journals require an abstract, and this is a logical place to begin reading the article. The abstract provides a brief overview of the article's contents, but because the information is a summary, you will not be able to judge the quality of the research or fully understand the theoretical basis, results, and implications without reading the full article. Some journals now use a format called a structured abstract. If you read an article in a recent volume of the *Journal of Speech-Language-Hearing Research*, for example, you will see abstracts with headings such as *purpose*, *method*, *results*, and *conclusion*. The inclusion of headings of this type allows the reader to quickly identify the question(s) addressed in the study, typically in the purpose section, and the tentative answers, typically in the results and conclusion sections.

Once you have a broad understanding of the content of an article from reading the abstract, you have some idea that the article is one that is relevant to the topic you are researching. When you read the full article, I suggest you begin by identifying the research question or problem the author(s) were studying. In almost every research article you read, the research question(s) will appear in the paragraph or two immediately preceding the methods section. Sometimes you will see a series of actual questions listed in these paragraphs, although at other times you might read a statement of purpose. We will learn more about the various forms a research question or problem might take in Chapter 3. Once I know the question(s), I typically want to know the tentative answers next. Usually, in a well-written article, the authors will provide their interpretation of results and the possible answers to their research questions in the discussion section of the article. You might even find that the various questions or purposes of the research are clearly identified with subheadings in the discussion section. Once you have a general understanding of the research questions and possible answers, you are better prepared to read the full article. You will begin with the introduction and review of literature, and because you know the questions addressed in the study, you will have a good understanding why the author included certain topics in this review. As you read the methods section, you should be considering whether the way the researchers designed the study and the way they collected their data gives you confidence in the results of the study. A course in research methods should provide you with the knowledge you need to critically evaluate the articles you read. Finally, as you read the results section you will be able to judge how the numerical (quantitative) or verbal (qualitative) information reported there related to the interpretation and conclusions the authors presented in their discussion section.

Summary

As noted previously, research is an essential component of the professional practice of audiologists and speech-language pathologists. In your clinical practice you will utilize research on a regular basis because our professional research is the basis of our clinical practice from decisions about diagnosis and etiology to the approaches we use in treatment. Further, speech-language pathologists and audiologists might need to directly consult existing research on behalf of specific clients. This might occur when these professionals are required, perhaps by a funding agency, to document the effectiveness of a proposed treatment, or perhaps when the audiologist or speech-language pathologist needs additional information to decide on the best course of treatment.

Professionals who investigate the existing research literature on behalf of their clients or for their own professional development are acting in the role of a consumer of research. However, audiologists and speech-language pathologists working in clinical settings have many good reasons to participate in designing and conducting original research as well. Some of the skills associated with the diagnosis and treatment of communication disorders could transfer to the research setting. Professionals already engage in a scientific approach to problem-solving and regularly participate in observation and measurement of communication behaviors to document the effectiveness of their services (ASHA, 2003). Using these skills to generate new information for the professions could be a natural extension for some audiologists and speech-language pathologists. The motivation for such work might come from unanswered questions encountered in the clinical setting, as well as the need for research generated in an ecologically valid setting—the work settings of audiologists and speech-language pathologists. For some types of research, particularly assessment or treatment research, audiologists or speech-language pathologists working regularly in the field might obtain higher quality data because of their clinical skills and experience.

Review Questions

1. What is the first step in the scientific method?

2. What phrase refers to the use of scientific evidence to guide clinical decisions?
   a. systematic inquiry
   b. hypothesis testing

c. evidence-based practice

d. single subject research

3. Define cost effectiveness research.

4. Which of the following statements is true?

a. Empirical research involves the collection of new information through observation and measurement.

b. Empirical research involves a systematic review of existing information identified through a literature search.

5. In _____ research, data often includes verbal information such as a detailed description of behavior or a direct quote.

6. What are the two characteristics of a *true* experiment?

7. Match the following terms.

_____ independent variable

_____ dependent variable

_____ true experiment

a. outcome measure

b. random assignment

c. experimental manipulation

8. What kind of research includes case studies, surveys, studies of correlations between measures, or studies of preexisting differences?

9. Which of the following statements is true?

a. Single subject research is descriptive research in which a researcher provides a detailed report on the characteristics of an individual participant.

b. Single subject research is experimental research in which a participant experiences both the experimental and control conditions.

10. When reading a research report, where are you most likely to find the research questions or statement of purpose?

11. List the typical parts of a research report. When you start reading a research report, which part would you read first?

12. Which of the following statements is true?

a. Some of the skills associated with the diagnosis and treatment of communication disorders are similar to the skills required to conduct scientific research.

b. The skills required to conduct scientific research are entirely different from the skills associated with the diagnosis and treatment of communication disorders.

References

American Speech-Language-Hearing Association. (2003). *Code of ethics* [Ethics]. Retrieved September 24, 2007, from http://www.asha. org/docs/html/ET2003-00166.html

American Speech-Language-Hearing Association. (2004). *Evidence-based practice in communication disorders: An introduction* [Technical report]. Retrieved January 3, 2007, from http://www.asha.org/docs/html/TR2004-00001.html

The American Speech-Language Hearing Association (2005). *Evidence-based practice in communication disorders* [Position Statement]. Retrieved August 24, 2008 http://www.asha.org

American Speech-Language-Hearing Association. (2007). *EBP compendium: All systematic reviews.* Retrieved June 30, 2008, from http://www.asha.org/members/ebp/compendium

Barnett, W. S. (2000). Economics of early childhood intervention. In J. P. Shonkoff & S. J. Meisels (Eds.), *Handbook of early childhood intervention* (2nd ed., pp. 589–610). Cambridge, UK: Cambridge University Press.

Gallagher, T. M. (2002). Evidence-based practice: Applications to speech-language pathology. *Perspectives on Language Learning and Education, 9*(1), 2–5.

Law, J., Garrett, Z., & Nye, C. (2004). The efficacy of treatment for children with developmental speech and language delay/disorder: A meta-analysis. *Journal of Speech, Language, and Hearing Research, 47*, 924–943.

MacNeil, J. R., Lui, C.-L., Stone, S., & Farrell, J. (2007). Evaluating families' satisfaction with early hearing detection and intervention services in Massachusetts. *American Journal of Audiology, 16*, 29–56.

Patten, M. L. (2007). *Understanding research methods: An overview of the essentials* (6th ed.). Glendale, CA: Pyrczak.

Peterson, H. A., & Marquardt, T. P. (1994). *Appraisal and diagnosis of speech and language disorders* (3rd ed.). Englewood Cliffs, NJ: Prentice Hall.

Robey, R. R. (1998). A meta-analysis of clinical outcomes in the treatment of aphasia. *Journal of Speech, Language, and Hearing Research, 41*, 172–187.

Sawyer, J., & Yairi, E. (2006). The effect of sample size on the assessment of stuttering severity. *American Journal of Speech-Language Pathology, 15*, 36–44.

Silverman, F. H. (1998). *Research design and evaluation in speech-language pathology and audiology: Asking and answering questions* (4th ed.). Englewood Cliffs, NJ: Prentice Hall.

Skahan, S. M., Watson, M., & Lof, G. L. (2007). Speech-language pathologists' assessment practices for children with suspected speech sound disorders: Results of a national survey. *American Journal of Speech-Language Pathology, 16*, 246–259.

Spielman, J., Ramig, L. O., Mahler, L., Halpern, A., & Gavin, W. J. (2007). Effects of an extended version of the Lee Silverman Voice Treatment on voice and speech in Parkinson's disease. *American Journal of Speech-Language Pathology, 16*, 95–107.

Stierwalt, J. A. G., & Youmans, S. R. (2007). Tongue measures in individuals with normal and impaired swallowing. *American Journal of Speech-Language Pathology, 16*, 148–156.

Taylor, R. S., Paisley, S., & Davis, A. (2001). Systematic review of the clinical and cost effectiveness of digital hearing aids. *British Journal of Audiology, 35*(5), 271–288.

Trochim, W. M. K., & Donnelly, J. P. (2007). *The research methods knowledge base* (3rd ed.). Mason, OH: Thomson Custom.

Turner-Stokes, L., Disler, P. B., Nair, A., & Wade, D. T. (2005). Multi-disciplinary rehabilitation for acquired brain injury in adults of working age. *Cochrane Database of Systematic Reviews*, Issue 3. Art. No.: CD004170.DOI: 10.1002/14651858.CD004170.pub2.

van Kleeck, A., Vander Woude, J., & Hammett, L. (2006). Fostering literal and inferential language skills in head start preschoolers with language impairment using scripted book-sharing discussions. *American Journal of Speech-Language Pathology, 15*, 85–95.

Yiu, E. M-L., Verdolini, K., & Chow, L. P. Y. (2005). Electromyographic study of motor learning for a voice production task. *Journal of Speech, Language, and Hearing Research, 48*, 1254–1268.

CHAPTER 2

Ethical Considerations

Regardless of their work setting, audiologists and speech-language pathologists who consider carrying out an original research project have many questions and concerns. They might wonder if they have sufficient time to conduct the research, the skills to perform certain procedures, or the equipment and other resources needed for the project. Hopefully, one of their foremost concerns will be their ability to conduct the research in an ethical manner. When you behave in an ethical way, you act according to a set of moral standards that characterize appropriate conduct. Professionals in fields such as audiology and speech-language pathology have formal codes established by national and state organizations (e.g., American Speech-Language-Hearing Association, American Academy of Audiologists, the various state speech-language-hearing associations). Certainly, there are ethical standards that guide us through all phases of a research project from identifying a problem and formulating research questions, to conducting the research and data gathering, to the eventual dissemination and possibly publication of your findings.

Protection of Human Participants

One of the primary considerations in the ethical conduct of research is protecting the well-being of the persons who participate in that research. Policies and regulations that guide us in protecting participants in research have been established by federal agencies, professional associations, as well as at the local level. Agencies that receive federal funds for research, such as universities, major medical centers, and school districts, need to have guidelines in place for the ethical conduct of research. Some of the essential protections for human participants include the requirement that participation be voluntary and not coerced, that researchers safeguard participants from any psychological or physical harm, that participants have an appropriate amount of information about the nature and purpose of the research before they are asked to take part (i.e., the notion of *informed consent*), that researchers take steps to maintain confidentiality and protect their participants' privacy, and finally, that participants understand they have a right to discontinue participation in the research study, even if they previously gave their consent.

These protections for research participants have their roots in a pioneering federal document, the Belmont Report, from the U.S. Department of Health and Human Services (National Commission, 1979). The authors of the Belmont Report identified three basic principles of culturally acceptable behavior that were also very important in the conduct of research. These included "respect of persons, beneficence and justice" (National Commission, 1979, Part B: Basic Ethical Principles, paragraph 1). Respect of persons involves recognizing persons' ability to make their own choices and decisions. Potential participants in research are able to make informed decisions when researchers provide them with sufficient information about the study and when their decision to participate is completely voluntary. For such a decision to be truly voluntary, potential participants should not be coerced or enticed with rewards they could only earn by participating in the research. For example, university professors sometimes encourage their students to participate in research by providing extra credit toward a better course grade. This might be an inappropriate enticement unless the professor also provides alternate ways, unrelated to research participation, for students to earn the extra credit. Similarly, provision of audiology and speech-language pathology services to individuals with speech, language, or hearing disorders should never be contingent on the person's agreeing to participate in research. Some persons, such as children or persons with cognitive disabilities, might have difficulty making an informed decision about their participation. Researchers need to pro-

vide special protections to such persons. This does not mean that children or persons with disabilities cannot participate in research, but it does mean that researchers need to consider consent more broadly and obtain permission from parents, guardians, or significant others.

The principle of *beneficence* relates to researchers' obligation to protect the well-being of the persons who participate in a study. In proposing a study, researchers consider whether they are providing a direct benefit to the participants or at least are obtaining information that contributes to the good of society. The former might occur when a researcher finds that a new treatment is more effective than the traditional, accepted practice. The latter might occur in a study that uncovers information about the nature of a disorder or principles of behavior change that will contribute to more effective treatment in the future. An essential requirement of beneficence in research is to protect participants from harm. You might recognize the dictum, "Above all, do no harm," as a statement from the oath that guides physicians and other medical professionals.[1] Researchers too must plan their studies in such a way that they expect to "do no harm" to their participants (National Commission, 1979). However, the nature of research is to investigate the unknown or the untried, and researchers might not be able to anticipate the potential harm a new experimental procedure could do. Thus, a second guideline for researchers is to "maximize possible benefits and minimize possible harms" (National Commission, 1979, Part B: Basic Ethical Principles, paragraph 7).

Let's consider some examples of the ways that researchers might conduct a study to minimize possible harms, even unantici-

---

[1]The statement, "Above all, do no harm," is often attributed to the Hippocratic Oath. Although Hippocrates wrote about similar concepts, this statement is not actually found in the Hippocratic Oath (C. M. Smith, 2005).

pated ones. You might be familiar with the studies that major pharmaceutical companies conduct to test the effectiveness of new drugs. The various news reporting agencies and news Web sites often include information about these "drug trials." When researchers undertake such a study they might not be able to anticipate the negative side effects of a new drug. However, to minimize the risk for participants they would carefully monitor each individual's health through periodic medical examinations. They also would monitor the rate of occurrence of any adverse side effects in the group receiving the new drug and in a comparison, control group. Researchers have an obligation to reevaluate the advisability of continuing such a study if they observe an abnormally high rate of adverse side effects in their treatment group.

Audiologists and speech-language pathologists sometimes need to compare different treatment approaches as well. In speech-language pathology these types of studies often involve comparing a new treatment approach that the researcher expects to be more effective and a traditional approach with a long history. The researcher most likely concluded, based on indirect evidence such as theoretical principles or evidence of effectiveness in other fields, that the new treatment approach should be more effective than the traditional approaches. Examples of this type of comparison in audiology are studies with comparisons of different hearing aid technologies (Jenstad, Seewald, Cornelisse, & Shantz, 1999; Larson et al., 2000; Walden, Surr, Cord, Edwards, & Olson, 2000). In audiology and speech-language pathology the adverse side effects for participants are unlikely to be physical symptoms or life threatening. However, persons in the experimental group might receive a treatment that turned out to be less beneficial. For example, persons receiv-

ing an experimental, behavioral treatment for acquired motor speech disorders might have less improvement in accuracy of sound production or speech intelligibility than those receiving traditional treatment. Maybe persons with hearing loss who were fitted with an experimental hearing aid technology received lower scores on tests of speech discrimination and rated their user satisfaction lower than persons who were fitted with an established hearing aid technology. These would be unintended yet adverse effects of participating in the research. Audiologists and speech-language pathologists need to be aware of adverse effects such as these and carefully monitor the progress of the persons who participate in their research, as well as their reactions during any testing or measurement procedures.

Given concerns about protecting the well-being of persons who participate in research, you might wonder why governmental agencies, professional organizations, and universities, among others, encourage research endeavors. The reason is that the benefits of research usually outweigh the potential risks. In a sense, a researcher weighs the potential risks and benefits when deciding to conduct a study. When researchers have reasons to expect substantial benefits either for the individual participants or a societal group (e.g., persons with speech disorders, persons with hearing loss), then they have justification for conducting a study. The beneficial outcomes are obvious when the research results in a treatment for a previously untreatable illness or condition or greater improvement or more rapid improvement in speech, language, or hearing outcomes.

The concept of *justice* relates to the need to make equitable decisions regarding who is invited to participate in research. Sometimes individuals want to participate in research because a study might provide a personal benefit. This might be the case when a person has a disorder with no known treatment, and an experimental approach is the only option. Researchers' decisions to include or exclude particular groups should have a sound, scientific basis. The Code of Ethics of the American Speech-Language-Hearing Association (ASHA) specifically addresses this issue in the following statement: "Individuals shall not discriminate in the delivery of professional services or the conduct of research and scholarly activities on the basis of race or ethnicity, gender, age, religion, national origin, sexual orientation, or disability" (ASHA, 2003, Principles of Ethics I, C). On the other hand, research participants might experience some adverse effects during a study making involvement in the study less desirable. In the case of possible adverse effects, the burden of participating in the research should be shared equally. Ideally the persons who are invited to participate would come from the group of persons most likely to benefit from the research. If the benefits of the research will be widespread, then the participants should be drawn from a widely representative group.

Special Protections

Certain groups might be particularly vulnerable to exploitation in research and have been identified as needing special protections under federal law. These persons include prisoners, children, pregnant women and their fetuses, as well as persons with cognitive impairments (Centers for Disease Control and Prevention, 1997; U.S. Department of Health and Human Services [HHS], 2005). The need for special protections sometimes stems from concerns about persons' ability to make a free choice without undue influ-

ence. The case of persons in prison exemplifies why special protections might be needed. Persons in a prison are confined against their will and are living in circumstances where voluntary consent has little meaning. A prison environment usually provides limited opportunities to enrich one's life with respect to choices of entertainment, food, living space, and so forth. A person in prison might be overly influenced by the offer of a reward for participation in research and thus more likely than persons outside prison to volunteer to take part in a somewhat risky study. Further, some persons might view prisoners as owing a debt to society or as needing to make amends for the crimes that led to their incarceration. Because of this view, some might think it appropriate to ask prisoners to participate in research on behalf of society when the risks could be fairly substantial.

The special protections afforded persons in prison or other institutional settings, children, pregnant women and their fetuses, and persons with impairments that would affect their ability to make decisions encompass all three principles of human participant protection: respect of persons, beneficence, and justice. Respect for persons relates to providing individuals with appropriate information so they can make voluntary decisions about participation in research. Special protections related to informed decision making could include writing the consent document in language appropriate for the person's reading level, or providing appropriate, not excessive, rewards or incentives, because excessive rewards for participating might overly influence a person's judgment about the level of risk associated with a study. Other examples of special protections include limiting research with protected populations to studies that have minimal risk and a direct benefit. Who benefits from the research is an important consideration, and for special populations the expectation is that the research should directly benefit the individual or benefit a group of persons in similar circumstances.

Although we usually think of special protections in the context of shielding vulnerable populations from unwarranted risks, systematically excluding protected populations from research participation also could be detrimental to the individuals' well-being. Let's consider the situation of persons who have a medical condition that has no known treatment. An individual with an untreatable illness, whether relatively young, in prison, or cognitively impaired, might desire an opportunity to receive even an experimental treatment. Similarly, persons receiving audiology and speech-language pathology services might want to participate in a study that could lead to improved outcomes for themselves or others with similar communication disorders. Thus, the principle of justice means protecting persons from unfair burden in assuming the risks of research, while at the same time providing equitable opportunities to participate in beneficial research (Kiskaddon, 2005).

Historical Perspective

Recognition of the need to protect research participants emerged largely in response to reported instances of mistreatment or exploitation of persons in the conduct of scientific research. Sometimes the reports became public many years after the end of the studies, although in some instances the reports coincided with the need to stop research with unacceptable, negative consequences. Considering why some studies prompted strong public and professional reaction is worthwhile for persons who might be conducting their own original

research in the future. Three studies that are noteworthy, either because the study influenced current policies on protection of research participants or because the study triggered extensive discussion of research ethics, are the Tuskegee Syphilis Study (King, 1998), the hepatitis study at Willowbrook State School (Moreno, 1998; Nelson, 1998), and the Tudor study at the University of Iowa (Goldfarb, 2006; Tudor, 1939). In discussing each of these studies, our focus will be on learning the lessons each teaches regarding protection of research participants and specifically regarding respect for persons, beneficence, and justice. A thorough examination of the ethical issues associated with each study is beyond the scope of this chapter and has been addressed in other sources (Fairchild & Bayer, 1999; Goldfarb, 2006; Kahn, Mastroianni, & Sugarman, 1998).

The Tuskegee Syphilis Study is one of the most notorious research projects ever conducted in the United States. The study began in 1932 and continued for 40 years, ending in 1972 after the particulars of the study first became widely known and published in sources available to the general public (Centers for Disease Control and Prevention [CDC], n.d.; King, 1998). The study was conducted by the U.S. Public Health Service and its purpose was to study the effects of untreated syphilis. The participants in the study were 399 African American men with syphilis and 201 African American men without syphilis who served as controls (CDC, n.d.; King, 1998). The study is notorious because the way it was conducted violated the basic ethical principles of respect for persons, beneficence, and justice.

The participants in the study lived in an area of the country where many people lived in poverty. The researchers used an enticement of free medical checkups to encourage the men to sign up for the study. The men never were told the true nature of their disease, but rather were told that they had "bad blood" (Fairchild & Bayer, 1999); further, the men never were told about or offered a treatment that was available in 1930.[2] Even more alarming was, when penicillin became available as an effective treatment for syphilis in the mid 1940s, the researchers did not offer this new treatment nor inform their participants of it.

The Tuskegee Syphilis Study was conducted in a way that violated all three basic principles. Certainly the participants did not receive adequate information about their disease or its probable course at the outset of the study, violating the principle of respect for persons. Further, King (1998) noted that the offer of free medical examinations might be regarded as a coercive inducement for participation given the participants had almost no access to health care and lived in poverty. The principle of beneficence holds that researchers should take all steps possible to protect their participants from harm or to minimize potential harm that might unexpectedly emerge during a study. The researchers who conducted the Tuskegee Syphilis Study violated the principle of beneficence in withholding information about possible treatment at the beginning of the study, and particularly when they withheld information about the availability of penicillin and failed to offer this effective treatment for more than 25 years.

Recall that the principle of justice relates to making equitable decisions regarding who is invited to participate in research. Supposedly, the purpose of the Tuskegee Syphilis Study was to determine if untreated syphilis progressed differently in African American men. In such a case, the most appropriate participants would be men who

are African Americans. However, the way the researchers conducted the study, particularly the disregard for the health and well-being of participants over a long period of time, suggested exploitation of a vulnerable, devalued population. The participants were vulnerable because their poverty prevented them from seeking adequate health care. The participants may have been devalued because of their race. The way African American men were treated in the Tuskegee study reflected the racial discrimination that was prevalent in society when the study began (King, 1998). Thus, the questionable ethics of this study also involved violations of the principle of justice, particularly justice for racial minorities and persons living in poverty.

The Tuskegee Syphilis Study is often cited in discussions of research ethics (Kahn et al., 1998). According to Fairchild and Bayer (1999, p. 1), the study " . . . has come to symbolize the most egregious abuse on the part of medical researchers." The study participants and their families were eventually awarded $10 million in an out-of-court settlement that followed their 1973 class-action lawsuit, and reaction to the study helped shape current national policies regarding the protection of research participants (National Commission, 1979).

Another example often cited in discussions of protection of research participants is a series of studies of hepatitis infection that took place at the Willowbrook State School in New York (Nelson, 1998). The study took place from 1955 through the early 1970s. This study is notable for at least two reasons. First, the participants in the study were children with developmental disabilities who were residents at the Wil-

---

[2]According to a document available on the CDC (n.d.) Web site, a treatment with mercury and bismuth was available by 1932. This treatment had a low cure rate and major toxic side effects; however, participants should have received information about this treatment option and been able to make a decision about seeking this option on their own.

lowbrook State School. Second, the study involved deliberately infecting the children with a strain of the hepatitis virus. The researchers justified exposing children to the virus on the basis that hepatitis infection was prevalent at the institute and most children who lived there were eventually infected (Nelson, 1998). Rothman (1982), among others, disagreed with this contention, and suggested that the researchers were taking advantage of the poor living conditions at Willowbrook. Rothman suggested that Krugman and his colleagues could have made a positive difference for the children at Willowbrook had that been their focus rather than conducting their research.

The participants in the Willowbrook studies were perhaps among the most vulnerable in our society. They were children with disabilities who lived in an institutional environment. The discussion of the Willowbrook studies has focused on questions regarding how the researchers obtained consent for the children to participate, research with a particularly vulnerable population, and also whether or not the research provided any benefit to participants (Diekma, 2006; Freedman, 2001; Goldby, 1971; Krugman, 1971; Moreno, 1998; Nelson, 1998; Ramsey, 2002).

As noted previously, one of the controversies associated with the Willowbrook studies centered on respect for persons and informed consent. The researchers did obtain permission from the children's parents before enrolling them in the study. Diekma (2006) noted the researchers employed a comprehensive consent process that included a meeting with a social worker as well as a group meeting where parents learned about the research. As thorough as this process was, however, at least two issues emerged that drew serious criticism. First, some authors pointed out that infor-

mation provided the parents was incomplete or even misleading (Freedman, 2001). Rothman (1982) noted that information in the consent form might have led parents to think their children would receive a vaccination for the virus, although the actual intent of the study was to infect children with a strain of the hepatitis virus under controlled conditions. Further, some parents received a letter regarding the study shortly after learning that the institution had no openings currently and their child would be placed on a waiting list. Thus, they were offered an earlier placement in the institution that was contingent on their child's participation in the research (Ramsey, 2002). For parents who wanted their children placed in the institution, this offer certainly could be coercive and have undue influence on their decision to let their children participate in the research.

Another controversy often discussed is whether or not children ever should be a part of a nontherapeutic research (Bartholome, 1978; Jonsen, 2006; Ramsey, 1978; Ramsey, 2002), and whether or not the Willowbrook research provided any medical benefits to the participants (Goldby, 1971; Krugman, 1971). Diekma (2006) summarized current thinking on children's participation in research as follows:

> Because children represent a vulnerable subject population, their involvement in research can be justified only if the level of risk entailed in the research is very low, or if there is the potential for direct benefit to the child by participating in the research project. (p. S7)

With regard to the Willowbrook studies, the deliberate infection of children with the hepatitis virus certainly posed more than minimal risk. Therefore, the debate regarding these studies focused on the possibility that the research offered some therapeutic benefit for the children who participated. The researchers who conducted the studies argued that the risks to the children in the studies were not more than that of any child living at Willowbrook, and perhaps less (Krugman, 1971). The rate of hepatitis infection at the institution was very high, and the children had a high probability of infection once they entered the institution. The research participants were infected under controlled circumstances and lived in a special ward that provided better medical care and living conditions. Further, Krugman (1971) maintained that children with hepatitis experience a relatively mild illness and afterwards would have some immunity, at least for one particular strain of the hepatitis virus. Krugman emphasized that the intent of the research was to obtain information needed to control the hepatitis problem at the institution and, thus, would directly benefit the children who lived at Willowbrook.

Critics of the Willowbrook studies argued that appealing to the poor conditions at the institution, which led to a high rate of hepatitis infection, was a weak defense for the research (Goldby, 1971; Rothman, 1982). Rothman (1982) noted that a treatment that was known to lessen the illness associated with hepatitis infection, inoculation with gamma globulin, was available, but this treatment was withheld from the children in the study. Further, Rothman asserted that the high rate of hepatitis infection at the institution was due to poor living conditions and the researchers could have taken steps to improve those conditions. The controversy over the Willowbrook studies was never fully resolved (Diekma, 2006; Jonsen, 2006). An important unanswered question is if research of this type would have been approved at an institution that served adults or children who were free of disabilities (Nelson, 1998; Ramsey, 2002).

The Willowbrook studies were conducted with the full knowledge of several medical boards and committees that reviewed the studies ahead of time and provided oversight for the research (Nelson, 1998). Thus, both the researchers who conducted the study as well as those responsible for administration of the school and oversight of the research could be the focus of criticism. Eventually, the Willowbrook State School was involved in legal action that sought to improve conditions at the school and to move residents out of this large institutional environment (Grossman, 1987).

The final research example we will consider is a study conducted in 1939 at the University of Iowa by a graduate student, Mary Tudor, under the direction of Dr. Wendell Johnson (Goldfarb, 2006; Tudor, 1939). In comparison to the Tuskegee and Willowbrook studies, Tudor's study was relatively unknown and had little impact on current national policy regarding the protection of participants in research. The study had few participants, 22 children in total, only 6 of whom prompted concerns about the conduct of the study. The study is interesting in communication sciences and disorders because Wendell Johnson was one of the pioneers in the field of speech-language pathology (Goldfarb, 2006), and also because the study has lessons to teach regarding our current thinking about treatment of child participants in research. The way the study was first reported in the popular press also teaches lessons regarding accurate, careful dissemination of information (Yairi, 2006).

The purpose of Tudor's research was to study how verbal labeling affected children's speech fluency (Tudor, 1939; Yairi, 2006). The participants in the study were

22 children who were residents at the Iowa Soldiers and Sailors Orphans' Home. Ten of the children were considered stutterers before the study, and 12 were children who were considered normal speakers.[3] To test the effects of verbal labeling, Tudor met with the children several times over a 5-month period. During these meetings she spoke to the children in different ways. Half of the children who stuttered received positive comments suggesting that their speech was fine, and half of the children with normal speech received highly negative comments suggesting they were having trouble speaking, that they had the signs of stuttering, and that they should try not to stutter (Silverman, 1988[4]; Yairi, 2006). Tudor also gave the staff at the children's home information about the children's "diagnoses." With respect to the original research questions, Tudor's results were unremarkable. The procedures produced no consistent changes in the fluency levels of the participants. However, Tudor's research notes suggested that some of the children in the normal speaking group who were subjected to negative comments changed in other ways. For example, they showed signs of being reluctant or self-conscious about speaking, and some commented on having difficulty with speaking (Reynolds, 2006; Tudor, 1939).

The six children who Tudor subjected to negative comments were at the center of a controversy that emerged more than 60 years later, after the publication of an article about the study in the *San Jose Mercury News* (Goldfarb, 2006). The sensationalized way the study was reported is one reason it became briefly infamous when it surfaced in 2001. The newspaper article suggested the researchers set out to turn children into stutterers, and Wendell Johnson, in an effort to avoid criticism, concealed the results of the study and never published it. Further, the study had a colorful nickname, the "monster" study,[5] a label taken from a 1988 *Journal of Fluency Disorders* article (Silverman, 1988). The information in the popular press misrepresented the actual research questions Tudor and Johnson investigated, as well as the nature of their findings.[6]

For professionals in the field of communication sciences and disorders, who inevitably viewed the Tudor study through the lens of contemporary thinking about protection of research participants and professional ethics, learning about the Tudor study was disturbing. Clearly this study would not be conducted as originally designed under current research guidelines and policies (Schwartz, 2006; Yairi, 2006). Considering why professional and public reaction to the study was so strong could help us better understand current thinking about children's participation in research. Because of their vulnerability, children are

---

[3]Yairi (2006) discussed the Tudor study in detail. He noted that the fluency levels among the children regarded as stutterers and those regarded as normal speakers were not clearly distinct and the two groups overlapped to a considerable degree.

[4]For readers who are interested in the exact nature of Tudor's comments, Silverman (1988) provides a few lengthy excerpts from the thesis manuscript.

[5]In a 1988 article Silverman stated that Tudor's study " . . . was labeled the 'monster' study by some of the persons who were associated with the Stuttering Research Program at the University of Iowa during the 1940s and 1950s and who knew of its existence" (p. 225). However, Silverman never elaborated on the exact reasons these individuals had for using this label.

[6]Ambrose and Yairi (2002) and Yairi (2006) provided a scholarly critique of Tudor's study, and Yairi (2006) also discussed how the study was reported in the popular press.

regarded as needing special protections in research. Generally, researchers accept that the types of studies children participate in should be limited to those with minimal risks or those that might provide a direct, personal benefit. In the Tudor study only the children who already stuttered who received positive verbal comments stood to benefit from the research. Because the concept of risk encompasses psychological as well as physical risks, the children with normal speech who received negative verbal comments were exposed to some degree of risk. Some authors have argued that, when research involves more than minimal risks, parents or guardians should not be able to give consent for their children to participate (Ramsey, 1978; Ramsey, 2002).

The Tudor study also had features that illustrate the need to consider beneficence and justice in the design of research. With regard to beneficence, the possibility that either Tudor or Johnson intended to cause any harm to the children seems remote (Yairi, 2006). However, Tudor's research notes, as well as statements from the participants more than 60 years later, suggested some unintentional harm did occur (Reynolds, 2006). Tudor intended to study changes in the children's fluency, but what she observed were general communication changes associated with being reluctant or self-conscious about speaking. One lesson researchers can learn from this is to be observant of unintended changes in participant behavior, as Tudor was, but also to be willing to modify or even stop research that is causing these changes. Rothman (1982) noted that sometimes researchers become overly focused on completing their studies. In such instances, researchers might overlook the possible negative effects the research procedures are having on their participants.

With regard to justice, the fact that the children were residents of an institution for orphaned or abandoned children was noteworthy. Historically, persons who resided in institutions of various types were exploited in research, leading to guidelines identifying prisoners and persons in other institutions as uniquely vulnerable populations in need of special protections (Moreno, 1998; National Commission, 1979). Ideally, the benefits and risks of research should be shared in an equitable way. The questions addressed in Tudor's study, regarding the effects of verbal labeling on dysfluency, were questions that were important to children and parents in general, not just to children living in a home for orphans. Reportedly, Tudor and Johnson conducted their study at the orphanage because the University of Iowa had a prior research relationship with the institution (Reynolds, 2006). As a sample of "convenience," the six children in Tudor's research took on more than their fair share of risk when they participated in the study. Current research guidelines, such as those for persons in prison (HHS, 2005), suggest that permissible research would address questions unique to the institutional environment including the conditions that led to imprisonment, or providing a personal benefit to the participants, such as an opportunity to receive new, more effective treatment for an illness.

Although the Tudor study reflected the research ethics of its time, it raised questions of respect for person, beneficence, as well as justice when it became widely known over 60 years later. In 2002 a lawsuit was brought against the State of Iowa on behalf of the three surviving participants and the estates of three other participants (Heldt, 2007). These were the individuals, who as 6- to 15-year-old children, were the targets of Tudor's attempts to increase dysfluency. In August 2007, the State of Iowa agreed to settle this lawsuit for $925,000 (Heldt, 2007).

Institutional Review Boards

One way that protections for research participants have been enhanced is through the process of institutional review (Penslar, 1993). Organizations such as universities, medical research facilities, and other research institutions that conduct research under federal regulations are required to provide institutional oversight through the process of an *institutional review board* (IRB). The role of an IRB is to evaluate proposed studies before the researchers begin collecting data. Researchers provide the IRB with a description of their proposed study, including information about the research design, participants, procedures, participant recruitment, and informed consent. The IRB reviews these materials and determines if the study adheres to guidelines associated with respect for persons, beneficence, and justice. A particular role of the IRB is to conduct a risk/benefit analysis of the proposed research to determine if risks to participants are minimal or justifiable based on potential benefits to the participants themselves or to society (Penslar, 1993). Although individual researchers still should endeavor to design projects that adhere to federal guidelines as well as the ethical standards of their professional associations, the IRB provides an opportunity for researchers to receive guidance from a qualified panel and an additional layer of protection for potential research participants.

Although protection of human participants in research is one of the researcher's primary ethical responsibilities, it is not the only one. Other issues to consider involve assigning credit for intellectual effort, accurate attribution of ideas and citing sources, accuracy and honesty in reporting information, potential conflicts of interest, and maintaining confidentiality and privacy of information (American Psychological Association [APA], 2002; ASHA, 2003; D. Smith, 2003). The final sections of this chapter address each of these topics in turn.

Credit for Intellectual Effort

In a way, receiving credit for intellectual effort relates to researchers' sense of ownership and desire to earn rewards for their ideas. When a researcher works alone on a project, identifying who "owns" and receives credit for a study is fairly straightforward. However, researchers often work together in teams or are students working under the direction of a faculty adviser (D. Smith, 2003). Ideally, in such instances the individuals involved should discuss their perceptions of their roles and contributions early in the planning process. That way the research team can avoid any misunderstanding before they reach a critical point in the project. One of the major rewards for conducting research is having an opportunity to present or publish the results of the study. D. Smith (2003) noted that this particular form of reward has taken on special importance in some research settings, such as universities, where decisions about retention and promotion are partially based on how much a person has published. Smith characterizes this as a " . . . competitive 'publish or perish' mindset" (2003, p. 56). Conversely, some researchers, particularly those in senior positions who have a long record of publication, might be tempted to be very generous in sharing credit for research. However, in sharing the rewards of their work, researchers need to be careful to give credit only to those who have made an actual contribution and also to consider the significance of that contribution (APA, 2002; ASHA, 2003; D. Smith, 2003). Sometimes the appropriate form of credit might be an acknowledgement rather than authorship; however, when the individual made an important contribution, she should be included as one of the authors. According to Smith (2003, p. 56), when researchers " . . . contribute substantively to the conceptualization, design, execution, analysis or interpretation of the research reported, they should be listed as authors."

Attribution of Ideas

Another way the researchers receive credit for their work is when others cite it in their own writing. Researchers publish the results of their studies because they hope to influence the work of other researchers and to inspire new projects. As writers we need to acknowledge the original author whenever we include an idea in our work that comes from another source. The ASHA Code of Ethics includes the following statement on the use of others' work: "Individuals shall reference the source when using other persons' ideas, research, presentations, or products in written, oral, or any other media presentation or summary" (ASHA, 2003, Principles of Ethics IV, E). When writers use information from another source they often paraphrase it in their own words. Even when paraphrasing information you still should give credit to the original source. Beginning professional writers sometimes ask the question, "How do I know when to attribute information to a particular source?"

One possible answer is to consider if the information is common knowledge in the profession or unique to a particular source. It is essential to cite the source when the information you use reflects the special expertise of another author. Sometimes the same information might be found in several sources but still reflects the special expertise of those authors. For example, several authors who are experts on the topic of specific language impairment might define this term in similar ways; or authors who are experts on the topic of central auditory processing disorders might provide similar guidance regarding appropriate testing. In instances of this type, you should cite all of the sources for the information. Certainly, deciding whether information is common knowledge or reflects some special expertise is a subjective judgment. However, if you have any doubt, you should include your sources. Providing a few citations that were unnecessary is better than mistakenly taking credit for another person's ideas.

Another issue for beginning writers is distinguishing between an accurate paraphrase of another author's work and plagiarism. Students sometimes ask, "How much do I need to change the original author's work to avoid plagiarism?" The key to avoiding plagiarism and generating your own paraphrase is not to start with statements written by another author. Small modifications such as changing a few words in a sentence by using synonyms, putting the key phrases in a different order, changing from present to past tense, and so forth are all writing strategies to avoid. A better strategy is to begin by trying to understand a passage when you read it (Purdue University Online Writing Lab [OWL], 2007; UW-Madison Writing Center, 2006). Once you are comfortable with your understanding, write down some notes using short phrases or words that are your own. Later you can use these notes to generate a summary or paraphrase of the information.[7] The Purdue OWL suggested several steps to generate an accurate paraphrase in your own words. The suggestions included reading for comprehension even if you have to read a passage more than once, writing your notes or paraphrase from memory, rereading the original text and comparing it to your paraphrase to check your accuracy, identifying any unique terms or phrases that you took directly from the source by using quotation marks, and including the information you will need for an accurate citation with your notes.

A final point to address in your writing is when and how often to use direct quotes. A direct quote from the original author could be the best approach when you find yourself struggling to restate or paraphrase a point. A direct quote is preferable to making small changes in the original and risking plagiarism. Similarly, a direct quote is preferable when the original sentence or passage is particularly clear; and any paraphrase, even a well-written one, weakens the line of reasoning. Writers use direct quotes for other reasons as well. For example, a writer might choose a direct quote from a recognized expert in a field to add credibility to an argument, or a writer might use a direct quote when presenting an opinion that is contrary to the writer's own point of view (Purdue OWL, 2006). A key point when using a direct quote is to identify it with quotation marks for a shorter quote or use an indented block style for longer quotes (APA, 2005). Usually you also should include the page number where you found the quoted statement.

Accuracy in Reporting Information

Another aspect of research ethics is the accurate representation of findings in your reports and presentations. Authors sometimes inadvertently report inaccurate findings due to mistakes in collecting, entering, or analyzing their results. This is not the kind of misrepresentation that raises ethical concerns. Usually, when authors discover they made an inadvertent error, they make sure their publisher or an appropriate organization issues a correction. The kind of misrepresentation that raises ethical concerns is the deliberate misrepresentation of results (Reis, 2001). Changing a number or two to increase the significance of your findings, reporting findings that you fabricated, or representing another person's findings as your own are all examples of deliberate misrepresentation of information. Any form of deliberate misrepresentation is considered *scientific misconduct* and, depending on the nature of the deception, could lead to serious penalties (Kintisch, 2005). Certainly, deliberate misrepresentation is a violation of the codes that define scientific and professional ethics (APA, 2002; ASHA, 2003).

Given the possibility of facing serious penalties as well as professional embarrassment, you might wonder why any researcher would risk falsifying information in her presentations and publications. One reason might be to increase the likelihood of receiving research funding (Kintisch, 2005). The competition for research grants is highly

---

[7]Any readers who are uncomfortable with their ability to write in their own words could benefit from a simple Internet search using terms such as *paraphrase* or *avoiding plagiarism*. You will find resources at several university Web sites such as the Purdue OWL and the Writing Center at the University of Wisconsin–Madison. These resources include examples as well as practice items.

intense and receiving this type of funding is very important in some fields of study and work settings. Another reason researchers might be tempted to falsify data is to increase the possibility of getting a study published. If you perused the research publications in any field, including audiology and speech-language pathology, you would learn that the vast majority of published research involves significant findings. In many universities and other research settings, professional prestige is based to a large degree on having a strong track record of publication. For at least some researchers, the desire for grant funding and professional recognition overpowers their sense of professional ethics (Brainerd, 2000; Reis, 2001). Further, identifying instances of misrepresentation of findings is very difficult in the typical review process for research publications and presentations (Kintisch, 2005). Rather, scientific misconduct usually is uncovered when it is reported by those who observed it, frequently research colleagues or even students (Couzin, 2006).

Avoiding Conflicts of Interest

Individuals face the possibility of a conflict of interest when they perform more than one role. Sometimes the obligations of one role are at odds with the responsibilities of other roles. Researchers who perform clinical research, such as audiologists and speech-language pathologists who study the nature, assessment, and treatment of speech-language-hearing disorders, might experience such conflicts. For example, researchers might want to investigate the effectiveness of a new treatment approach that, in theory, should be stronger than treatment approaches currently used in the field. However, the researchers cannot be certain the new treatment is better until

they gather some evidence. Professionals in this situation must balance their desire to investigate the new treatment with their desire to provide known, effective treatment to their clients with communication disorders. If they lean too heavily toward their research role, they might try experimental treatments with clients that have little chance of success. However, if they lean too heavily toward their clinician role, they might miss opportunities to advance the professions through research that leads to more effective clinical procedures.

Another point when speech-language pathologists and audiologists in the dual roles of researchers and clinicians might experience conflicts of interest is in recruiting participants for their studies. If researchers recruit participants from among persons they serve clinically, they must be equally supportive of their clients' decisions, whether the clients agree to participate or decline to participate in any studies. The fact that a client was or was not a research participant should have no impact on the quality of speech-language or audiology services they receive. Keeping the clinician-client and researcher-participant roles separated is particularly challenging, because clients might assume their clinical services might be negatively affected. That is, the client's consent to participate might be coerced, through fear of losing access to treatment, even if that never was the researcher's intention. Perhaps the best way to manage this conflict between clinician and researcher roles is to ask a third party to manage the process of participant informed consent. That way the clinician-researchers avoid talking directly to any of their clients about participating in their research.

Another example of a conflict of interest is a conflict between the roles of researcher and product developer. Perhaps a speech-language pathologist or audiologist developed a product she thinks will improve assessment or treatment of communication disorders. One factor potential purchasers of this product might consider is whether or not the new product is superior to the assessment and treatment tools they already use. If the product developers designed and conducted research to demonstrate its superiority, this might constitute a conflict of interest. What would happen if the researcher-developers found evidence that existing assessment or treatment products were more effective? They might be tempted to conceal that evidence or to redesign their study in hopes of obtaining more favorable results. In this case the desire of the developers to market their product might be at odds with conducting and accurately reporting the results of their research. Ideally, product developers should recruit independent researchers to evaluate the superiority of new products or conduct research on new assessment and treatment instruments before making plans to market those instruments.

D. Smith (2003) identified another possible conflict of interest, a conflict between the roles of instructor and researcher. One example of this is common in psychology when course instructors recruit their students to participate in research projects (Smith, 2003). In some courses, participating in research is a course requirement; in others students receive extra credit for participating in research. Instructors should be careful to provide students who choose not to participate in research with alternative ways to earn course or extra credit. Otherwise, instructors could be perceived as coercing their students into participating in research. The principles of informed consent include the requirement that participants make their decision to participate free of coercion. Instructor-researchers might face another conflict of interest when the students in their courses also work as their research assistants. In this case, researchers need to be careful about how much work they ask their assistants to do or how they set up their schedules. Students who are research assistants might agree to a work overload or a burdensome work schedule because they think refusing could have a negative impact on their course grade (Smith, 2003). Instructor-researchers should be aware of this potential conflict, carefully monitor the hours their research assistants work, and encourage their assistants to communicate with them about workload issues.

Confidentiality and Privacy

A final issue in research ethics is the need for researchers to maintain the confidentiality and privacy of information they obtain from research participants (APA, 2002; ASHA, 2003). Some basic procedures to ensure confidentiality include using identification codes rather than participants' names on all research documents; avoiding any mention of participants' names in any publications or presentations; and maintaining all documents, particularly consent forms that include identifying information, in a secure location. D. Smith (2003) identified several other concerns associated with confidentiality and privacy. For example, researchers need to consider the extent to which they might want to share their data before they obtain informed consent from their participants. Unless participants know that other researchers might examine and use their responses when they sign the consent form, only the original research team should typically have access to the data. Smith also noted that researchers need to make sure others cannot overhear them when discussing participants and to be aware of computer security issues, particularly those associated with networked computers. Some research might involve medical records covered under the Health Insurance Portability and Accountability Act ([HIPAA]; HHS, 2003). When this is the case researchers must adhere to HIPAA guidelines for assuring privacy and security of personal medical records (ASHA, 2007).

Data collection approaches that use video or audiotapes of participants present special concerns for maintaining confidentiality. Participants usually can be identified from a visual image and sometimes even from an audio recording. Sometimes participants make statements during recording that could identify them or comment in ways that could be embarrassing to them or their families. Thus, researchers need to be particularly careful about handling and storing participant recordings. Some precautions could include storing recordings in a secure laboratory or office, making sure research team members review recordings only in designated locations, and having a plan for how long to keep recordings and how to dispose of them at the end of the study.

Summary

In this chapter we reviewed a number of ethical considerations that guide all phases of research from initial planning to the final analysis and publication of our findings. Among the primary considerations is the need to protect the well-being of human participants. Both governmental regulations and professional ethics provide researchers with guidance on aspects of human subject participation such as informed consent, protecting the well-being of participants, maintaining confidentiality of participants' information, and assuring equitable distribution of the risks and rewards of research. Ethical conduct in research also encompasses other areas such as credit for intellectual effort in publishing research findings and when citing the work of others, maintaining high standards of accuracy and honesty in reporting findings, and recognizing potential conflicts of interest between the role of researcher and other professional roles.

Review Questions

1. What are the three basic principles of protection of human research participants identified in the Belmont Report?

2. Which of the three basic principles of protection of human participants means persons make their own, informed decisions about participating in research?

3. Given concerns about protecting the well-being of persons who participate in research, why do governmental agencies, professional organizations, and universities, among others, encourage research endeavors?

4. Which of the principles of protection of human participants means researchers need to make equitable decisions regarding who is invited to participate in research?

5. Identify two groups of research participants who receive special protections under federal law.

6. Provide an example of coercive or undue influence in recruiting participants for a research study.

7. Provide an example of a violation of the principle of beneficence in the conduct of a research study.

8. What are two reasons why present-day researchers feel that the Tudor (1939) study at the University of Iowa violated principles of human participant protection?

9. What do the letters IRB mean?

10. Match the following terms with their examples.

    _____ credit for intellectual effort
    _____ attribution of ideas
    _____ conflict of interest

    a. citing a source
    b. more than one role
    c. credit for authorship

11. Is it ever appropriate to use another author's words in your writing? Explain your answer.

12. What is plagiarism?

Learning Activities

1. The following Web sites have information on ethical conduct in research and protection of human participants. Visit one of these Web sites and explore some of the educational materials provided.
    a. American Speech-Language-Hearing Association Ethics Roundtable at: http://www.asha .org/about/ethics/roundtable/
    b. American Psychological Association—Human Research Protections at: http://www.apa .org/science/rcr/human.html
    c. American Psychological Association–Publication Practices and Responsible Authorship at: http://www.apa.org/science/rcr/ publication.html
    d. United States Department of Health and Human Services— Office for Human Research Protections at: http://www.hhs .gov/ohrp/

2. Alternately, conduct a Web search on a topic such as "protection of human participants" or "ethical conduct of research" and explore some of the information you retrieve.

References

Ambrose, N., & Yairi, E. (2002). The Tudor study: Data and ethics. *American Journal of Speech-Language Pathology, 11*(2), 190–203.

American Psychological Association. (2002). *Ethical principles of psychologists and code of conduct.* Retrieved November 17, 2007, from http://www.apa.org/ethics/code2002.pdf

American Psychological Association. (2005). *Concise rules of APA style.* Washington, DC: Author.

American Speech-Language-Hearing Association. (2003). *Code of ethics* [Ethics]. Retrieved September 24, 2007, from http://www.asha .org/docs/html/ET2003-00166.html

American Speech-Language-Hearing Association. (2007). *Guidelines for the responsible conduct of research: Ethics and the publica-*

tion process [Guidelines]. Retrieved August 24, 2008 from http://www.asha.org/docs/pdf/GL2007-00282.pdf

Bartholome, W. G. (1978). Central themes in the debate over the involvement of infants and children in biomedical research: A critical examination. In J. van Eys (Ed.), *Research on children: Medical imperatives, ethical quandaries, and legal constraints* (pp. 69–76). Baltimore: University Park Press.

Brainard, J. (2000). As U.S. releases new rules on scientific fraud, scholars debate how much and why it occurs [Electronic version]. *Chronicle of Higher Education, 47*(15). Retrieved November 20, 2007, from the EBSCO database. http://search.ebscohost.com/

Centers for Disease Control and Prevention. (1997). *CDC procedures for protection of human research participants.* Retrieved October 11, 2007, from http://www.cdc.gov/od/foia/manuals/procphrp.pdf

Centers for Disease Control and Prevention. (n.d.). *U.S. Public Health Service syphilis study at Tuskegee: The Tuskegee timeline.* Retrieved November 4, 2007, from http://www.cdc.gov/tuskegee/timeline.htm

Couzin, J. (2006, September). Scientific misconduct: Truth and consequences. *Science, 313*(5791), 1222–1226.

Diekma, D. S. (2006). Conducting ethical research in pediatrics: A brief historical overview and review of pediatric regulations [Electronic version]. *Journal of Pediatrics, 149*, S3–S11.

Fairchild, A. L., & Bayer, R. (1999, May 7). Uses and abuses of Tuskegee [Electronic version]. *Science, 284*(5416), 919–921.

Freedman, R. I. (2001). Ethical challenges in the conduct of research involving persons with mental retardation. *Mental Retardation, 39*(2), 130–141.

Goldby, S. (1971, April 10). Experiments at the Willowbrook State School [Letter to the editor]. *Lancet,1*(7702), 749.

Goldfarb, R. (Ed.). (2006). *Ethics: A case study from fluency.* San Diego, CA: Plural.

Grossman, J. B. (1987, Winter). Review: Beyond the Willowbrook Wars: The courts and insti-

tutional reform. *American Bar Foundation Research Journal, 12*(1), 249–259.

Heldt, D. (2007, August 17). Settlement to involved six UI 'Monster Study' plaintiffs. *The Gazette Online.* Retrieved November 17, 2007, from http://www.gazetteonline.com/apps/pbcs.dll/article?AID=/20070817/NEWS/70817017/1006/NEWS

Jenstad, L. M., Seewald, R. C., Cornelisse, L. E., & Shantz, J. (1999). Comparison of linear gain and wide dynamic range compression hearing aid circuits: Aided speech perception measures. *Ear and Hearing, 20*(2), 117–126.

Jonsen, A. R. (2006). Nontherapeutic research with children: The Ramsey versus McCormick debate. *Journal of Pediatrics, 149*, S12–S14.

Kahn, J. P., Mastroianni, A. C., & Sugarman, J. (Eds.). (1998). *Beyond consent: Seeking justice in research.* New York: Oxford University Press.

King, P. A. (1998). Race, justice, and research. In J. P. Kahn, A. C. Mastroianni, & J. Sugarman (Eds.), *Beyond consent: Seeking justice in research* (pp. 88–110). New York: Oxford University Press.

Kintisch, E. (2005, March). Scientific misconduct: Researcher faces prison for fraud in NIH grant applications and papers. *Science, 307*(5717), 1851.

Kiskaddon, S. H. (2005). Balancing access to participation in research and protection from risks: Applying the principle of justice [Electronic version]. *Journal of Nutrition, 135*, 929–932.

Krugman, S. (1971, May 8). Experiments at the Willowbrook State School [Letter to the editor]. *Lancet, 1*(7706),966–967.

Larson, V. D., Williams, D. W., Henderson, W. G., Luethke, L. E., Beck, L. B., Noffsinger, D., et al. (2000). Efficacy of 3 commonly used hearing aid circuits: A crossover trial [Electronic version]. *Journal of the American Medical Association, 284*(14), 1806–1813.

Moreno, J. D. (1998). Convenient and captive populations. In J. P. Kahn, A. C. Mastroianni, & J. Sugarman (Eds.), *Beyond consent: Seeking justice in research* (pp. 111–130). New York: Oxford University Press.

The National Commission for the Protection of Human Subjects of Biomedical and Behavioral Research. (1979). *The Belmont Report: Ethical Principles and Guidelines for the Protection of Human Subjects of Research.* U.S. Department of Health and Human Services. Retrieved September 22, 2007, from http://www.hhs.gov/ohrp/humansubjects/guidance/belmont.htm

Nelson, R. M. (1998). Children as research subjects. In J. P. Kahn, A. C. Mastroianni, & J. Sugarman (Eds.), *Beyond consent: Seeking justice in research* (pp. 47-66). New York: Oxford University Press.

Penslar, R. L. (Ed.). (1993). *Office of Human Research Protections (OHRP): IRB guidebook.* Retrieved November 17, 2007, from http://www.hhs.gov/ohrp/irb/irb_guidebook.htm

Purdue OWL. (2006, September 10). Quoting, paraphrasing, and summarizing. In *The Purdue Online Writing Lab.* Retrieved November 19, 2007, from http://owl.english.purdue.edu/owl/resource/563/01/

Purdue OWL. (2007, October 11). Paraphrase: Write it in your own words. In *The Purdue Online Writing Lab.* Retrieved November 19, 2007, from http://owl.english.purdue.edu/owl/resource/563/02/

Ramsey, P. (1978). Ethical dimensions of experimental research on children. In J. van Eys (Ed.), *Research on children: Medical imperatives, ethical quandaries, and legal constraints* (pp. 57-68). Baltimore: University Park Press.

Ramsey, P. (2002). *The patient as person: Explorations in medical ethics* (2nd ed.). New Haven, CT: Yale University Press.

Reis, R. M. (2001, July 20). Avoiding misconduct in your scientific research [Electronic version]. *Chronicle of Higher Education: Chronicle Careers.* Retrieved November 20, 2007, from http://chronicle.com/jobs/2001/07/2001072002c.htm

Reynolds, G. (2006). The stuttering doctor's "monster study." In R. Goldfarb (Ed.), *Ethics: A case study from fluency* (pp. 1-12). San Diego, CA: Plural.

Rothman, D. J. (1982). Were Tuskegee and Willowbrook "studies in nature?" *Hastings Center Report, 12*(2), 5-7.

Schwartz, R. G. (2006). Would today's IRB approve Tudor's study? Ethical considerations in conducting research involving children with communication disorders. In R. Goldfarb (Ed.), *Ethics: A case study from fluency* (pp. 83-96). San Diego, CA: Plural.

Silverman, F. H. (1988). The "monster" study. *Journal of Fluency Disorders, 13*, 225-231.

Smith, C. M. (2005). Origin and uses of *primum non nocere*—Above all, do no harm! *Journal of Clinical Pharmacology, 45*(4), 371-377.

Smith, D. (2003). Five principles for research ethics [Electronic version]. *Monitor on Psychology, 34*(1), 56.

Tudor, M. (1939). *An experimental study of the effect of evaluative labeling on speech fluency.* Unpublished master's thesis, University of Iowa, Iowa City.

U.S. Department of Health and Human Services, Office for Civil Rights. (2003, May). *Summary of the HIPAA privacy rule.* Retrieved August 24, 2008 from http://www.hhs.gov/ocr/privacysummary.pdf

U.S. Department of Health and Human Services. (2005). Protection of Human Subjects, 45 C.F.R. § 46. Retrieved September 28, 2007, from http://www.hhs.gov/ohrp/documents/OHRPRegulations.pdf

UW-Madison Writing Center. (2006). *Writer's handbook.* Retrieved November 19, 2007, from http://www.wisc.edu/writing/Handbook/index.html

Walden, B. E., Surr, R. K., Cord, M. T., Edwards, B., & Olson, L. (2000). Comparison of benefits provided by different hearing aid technologies. *Journal of the American Academy of Audiology, 11*(10), 540-560.

Yairi, E. (2006). The Tudor study and Wendell Johnson. In R. Goldfarb (Ed.), *Ethics: A case study from fluency* (pp. 35-62). San Diego, CA: Plural.

CHAPTER 3

Identifying and Formulating Research Questions

The starting point for most research projects is a problem that requires a solution or a question that needs an answer. Most of us have encountered problems or questions in our daily lives and engaged in some kind of investigation to find a solution to the problem or an answer to the question. Perhaps our automobile needed service and we had to find a reliable repair shop that would provide the service in a timely way and at a reasonable cost. Maybe we decided to upgrade to a new computer and wondered what seller would provide good service as well as a reasonable cost. Once we formulated our problem or question, we started to make some telephone calls, to talk with friends or family, to visit some retailers, and perhaps to consult some consumer publications. We began to gather information after identifying the problem or question. Similarly, researchers begin their process of inquiry by identifying some unknown information, which they express as a problem to resolve or as a question to answer. How researchers and consumers differ is in the precise way researchers state their questions, and in the process of preliminary investigation that researchers use to revise and refine their questions. Another type of question that audiologists and speech-language pathologists sometimes need to investigate is an evidence-based practice question. With these types of questions audiologists and speech-language pathologists investigate existing research to identify information that applies to persons they serve clinically. Although evidence-based practice questions might not lead to original research, generating a well-formed question is still an important consideration.

Identifying Important Questions

Sometimes students at the beginning of their professional training have asked how to find a viable research topic. Often these questions arise when students consider the requirements of their graduate programs, many of which require some type of research paper or offer the option of a research paper or thesis. When these questions are addressed to me, my advice always is to consider your professional interests. Although all audiologists and speech-language pathologists complete a broad program of study that encompasses all areas of the profession, most find certain areas of study more inherently interesting than others. Some examples to consider are the work setting you find most attractive (e.g., medical, school, private practice), any special interests you have in certain communication disorders (acquired cognitive or language disorders, phonological disorders in children, central auditory processing disorders), or an area of clinical practice you particularly enjoy (such as evaluation and diagnosis, counseling clients and their families, providing direct treatment, hearing aid fitting). Once you have identified a general focus for your research, a good strategy is to follow up by reading extensively in your particular areas of interest.[1]

Occasionally, speech-language pathologists and audiologists discover interesting questions even though they were not planning to conduct research. Rosenthal and Rosnow (2008) identified two forms of inspiration that could apply in clinical settings. The first example is finding inspiration for research from a case study. Perhaps a clinician encountered a particularly interesting case that inspired interest in research. Sometimes audiologists or speech-language pathologists encounter individuals in their clinical practice with unique needs that are not covered in the existing research. This might inspire a research interest to better understand these unique individuals and to provide them with more effective treatment. The second example is finding inspiration in contradictory or paradoxical situations or behaviors (Rosenthal & Rosnow, 2008). An example of this form of inspiration might involve encountering a client whose evaluation results are contradictory or who responds to treatment in a contrary manner.

Perhaps an audiologist has encountered several clients whose problems on certain perceptual tasks are much worse than would be predicted from other audiological test results, or a speech-language pathologist has identified several clients whose speech production errors in conversational speech are very different from those exhibited in single-word productions. Contradictions of this type might inspire clinicians to further explore the reasons why these clients behaved in unpredicted ways and eventually to even formulate research questions to investigate.

Silverman (1998) noted researchers also should consider several practical issues when they choose a question to investigate. Finding a question that is both interesting and practical is particularly important for students in graduate programs that might last only 2 to 4 years, depending on whether they are pursuing a master's degree, clinical doctorate, or research doctorate. Some of the practical considerations Silverman identified were how much time you have, whether or not you have the required skills, whether or not you have access to an appropriate group of participants, what equipment and facilities you have available, and what persons you need for support in conducting the research. Another consideration, particularly for students who are developing as investigators, is whether or not a mentor who is knowledgeable in your interest area is available to guide the research.

A few examples might clarify the challenge of finding a research question that is both motivating and practical. Some questions require that you gather information over a long period of time. One of the most impressive studies I have read was a study

---

[1]Another way to follow up on your professional interests is to find a mentor who conducts research in a similar area. In many scientific fields, graduate students work for several years in their mentors' laboratories before developing an independent line of research.

of the impact of participating in a preschool program on children's subsequent achievement in school and in life (Barnett, 2000). The researchers who conducted this study followed their participants from the time they were preschool children until they were young adults. The study yielded important information about the lasting effects of the preschool program but required the researchers to follow their participants for more than 15 years. Studies of this type are important for any field but are not practical to undertake in the typical time frame of a graduate program.

Some research questions might be practical only in research facilities associated with major medical centers. Perhaps the questions you find most interesting center on the development of speech perception in young children following a cochlear implant, neuroimaging studies of listeners' reactions to certain speech stimuli, or the genetic bases of speech, language, and hearing disorders. These are just a few examples of very interesting avenues of research that might be practical in only a few facilities where the researchers have access to experts from other professions, as well as expensive, highly specialized equipment.

A final factor to consider when choosing research questions is the importance to your field of study. Researchers in communication sciences and disorders might ask, "Would answering this question make a significant contribution to audiology, speech-language pathology, or speech and hearing science?" Judging the value of a research question is a subjective process, but you might find evidence in your reading to support your judgments. For example, an author who is highly respected in your field of study might have identified certain questions as worthwhile. When reading in your areas of interest, you might look for suggested research questions in review articles or in the discussion sections of research reports (Silverman, 1998). Often authors of research articles include suggestions for future research toward the end of their discussion sections. After discussing the results of existing research, authors will extend their discussion to address areas for further studies. Another way to identify significant questions is to consider questions that were posed and investigated but not answered in a definitive manner (Silverman, 1998). The original study might have weaknesses that you or other authors identified, such as a small sample size, inadequate outcome measures, or uncontrolled, extraneous variables that might have influenced the results. Perhaps the original study was well designed but left a number of related, unanswered questions. You might see ways to extend the original research in new directions. Consider some of the following possibilities:

1. Extend the study to a new research population such as a new age group, a different diagnostic group, or persons from a different linguistic or cultural background

2. Apply different outcome measures such as using measures from spontaneous speech if the original study used formal tests and/or measures from elicited speech samples

3. Address questions of social validity by determining the functional impact of observed changes for the participants or their families (Foster & Mash, 1999)

4. Change the stimuli used to elicit responses or the procedures for presenting stimuli to test whether findings are specific to certain stimuli or conditions

5. Change the setting in which an evaluation or treatment occurs to provide either a more naturalistic setting or a setting that more closely matches real clinical situations

6. Use up-to-date instrumentation in testing and analyzing participants' responses for approaches that might be dated

These are just a few suggestions for how one might modify an existing research approach to provide more complete and accurate answers to a question. The idea is to read existing research reports in an analytic way considering how ideas presented in an article or perhaps approaches to measurement and analysis might differ from what you have learned.

Perhaps the research question that was most interesting is an original idea that emerged from your reading or professional experiences. Silverman (1998, p. 61) referred to these as "questions that have not been formulated but should be." An original research question might emerge as an inspiration as we discussed previously. Another way original questions emerge is through researchers' familiarity with work in other fields of study. Researchers in communication sciences and disorders have found relevant ideas in many related disciplines, such as linguistics, psycholinguistics, developmental psychology, information processing, neuropsychology, and physiology, to name just a few. When supporting the importance of a question that emerged from work in other disciplines, researchers might include an explanation of the findings, procedures, theory, or principles and an explanation of their potential application in communication sciences and disorders. Explaining the importance of finding answers to particular questions generally involves making explicit the thought process that led you to formulate those questions, whether they emerged from a critical review of previous research, from reading research reports from other disciplines, or from your own professional experiences.

Readers might ask why it is important to investigate an important and relevant question, and why simply having a strong, personal interest in the question is not sufficient justification. A casual answer to such a question is that in some cases a strong personal interest in a question would be sufficient justification. Investigating relevant questions of broad interest in communication sciences and disorders is most important when researchers might want to publish their findings in the future, receive recognition for their efforts from peers or administrators, or possibly compete for financial support to conduct their research (Silverman, 1998). However, in most professional settings, a researcher must justify the importance of a proposed study to a review board before ever gathering data. Therefore, even if researchers were willing to forego future publication opportunities or other recognition, they still need a well-thought-out rationale for any questions they want to investigate.

Formulating Research Questions

Once researchers decide what questions they want to investigate, their next task is to frame the questions in an unambiguous way. When you read a well-written research question, you learn something about the design of the study as well as the kind of data the researchers obtained from their participants. Silverman (1998, p. 65) suggested that a well-written question is an answerable one that " . . . implicitly or explicitly (preferably the latter) specifies the observation or observations needed to answer it."

One of the first things to consider when writing a research question is how to specify what you are going to investigate. Usually interesting subjects to investigate are things that change or vary as the situation or circumstances change. Researchers use the term *variables* to refer to the phenomena they plan to observe. When studying a variable, researchers might study naturally occurring changes or manipulate the circumstances in an effort to create changes in a variable. The research is *nonexperimental* when the study centers on naturally occurring changes and *experimental* when the study centers on the researchers' manipulations to create changes.

Depending on the kind of the research, the question might specify both independent and dependent variables. *Independent variables* are the conditions or manipulations the researcher is interested in studying. In nonexperimental research the independent variables could include existing differences such as age groups, diagnostic categories, language backgrounds, and so forth. A common nonexperimental approach to research in communication sciences and disorders is to compare persons with communication disorders and those without communication disorders. For example, children with language impairments might be compared to children matched for chronological age and/or language age; or persons with moderate-to-severe hearing loss might be compared to persons with normal hearing. In experimental research the independent variables could include differences the researcher created by manipulating some circumstance. For example, the researcher might create two different versions of a task to determine how that manipulation affected the performance of the research participants, or the researcher might compare two different treatment programs to determine if either one is more effective.

The *dependent variables* in a study are the observations or measures a researcher obtains. For example, participants with communication disorders and those with normal communication might both complete a set of tests selected by the researchers. This type of study would be a nonexperimental comparison and the participants' scores on

the tests would be dependent variables. A similar example for an experimental study would involve administering the test before and after treatment. If researchers administered the test to two different treatment groups, they could compare the groups' scores. In this example, the test scores would be the dependent variable and the different treatment groups would be the independent variable. In experimental research the dependent variables are the researchers' outcome measures.

Another consideration in formulating a research question is the intent of the research. The way a research question is framed will depend on whether the researchers' aim is to describe persons or circumstances, to discover relationships between or among variables, or to identify differences between groups (Rosenthal & Rosnow, 2008). Consider the example of researchers who were interested in studying speech and language development in preschool children. The researchers decided to study several measures of speech development. Through their reading prior to designing a study, the researchers discovered several measures they thought were worthy of further investigation. An example of such a measure was the consonant-vowel (CV) ratio. The researchers considered a series of studies beginning with a descriptive approach, then a relational approach, and finally a study of differences. For these studies they framed their questions such as those posed in Table 3–1.

The sample questions in Table 3–1 were intended to illustrate how researchers might represent different types of studies, including descriptive, relational, and difference approaches. However, a researcher would need to refine these example questions before using them to guide the design of an investigation. We cover some of the criteria for developing well-formed research questions in a following section; but before

Table 3–1. Research questions that illustrate differences among descriptive, relational, and difference studies

Descriptive study:

1. What is the CV ratio for preschool children at ages 18 months, 24 months, 30 months, and 36 months?

Relational study:

2. What is the relationship between CV ratio and mean length of utterance in preschool children from ages 18 to 36 months?

Difference study—nonexperimental:

3. What is the difference in CV ratio between children with normal hearing and those with moderate-to-severe hearing loss at 24 months?

Difference study—experimental:

4. What is the difference in CV ratio for 24-month-old children with expressive language delay who participated in an 8-week intervention program compared to 24-month-old children with expressive language delay who received no intervention?

dealing with that issue, we consider various ways researchers might state the problem(s) they intend to investigate.

Ways to Formulate a Research Problem

One of the first steps in conducting a study is to clearly define the problem that the researchers intend to investigate. Although researchers frequently choose to state the problem or focus of their study in a research question or series of questions, research questions are not the only option. Some other approaches include formal hypotheses, a statement of purpose, or even conditional if-then statements.

Whether researchers use formal hypotheses, research questions, or a statement of purpose depends in part on the type of study they are conducting. For example, a researcher who is conducting a descriptive study is more likely to use research questions or a statement of purpose than formal hypotheses; a researcher who is conducting a relational or difference study, particularly one that involves statistical analyses, could use any approach including formal hypotheses, a statement of purpose, or research questions. For some studies the approaches to formulating a research problem are essentially interchangeable and the one you use is a matter of personal preference (Patten, 2007).

Traditionally, researchers conducting quantitative studies developed formal hypotheses when defining the problem they intended to investigate. A *hypothesis* is a formal statement of the predicted outcome of a study (Trochim & Donnelly, 2007). Actually, in stating the predicted outcome of a study, researchers often formulate two versions of their hypothesis. The first is called a *null hypothesis* and is sometimes abbreviated as H_0. The alternate hypothesis is sometimes called a *research hypothesis* and is abbreviated as H_1 (Patten, 2007).

A null hypothesis is stated in the negative and is based on the assumption that the results of a study will yield no significant differences between groups and/or no significant relationships among variables. In Table 3–2 some of the example questions presented in Table 3–1 are restated as null hypotheses.

The idea of a null hypothesis stems from quantitative studies in which researchers employ statistical procedures to evaluate their findings. The point of many statistical procedures is to test the viability of a null hypothesis. Based on their statistical findings, researchers will either *reject* the null hypothesis, meaning that the null hypothesis is not viable, or *fail to reject* the null hypothesis, meaning that the null hypothesis is viable. In a sense, the null hypothesis is a strategy for maintaining researchers' objectivity. A researcher states there is no relationship or no difference until or unless the data indicate otherwise. Researchers also have to be careful not to say that they have proven a null hypothesis is true. Failing to reject a null hypothesis is not the same thing as concluding or proving that two variables are not related, or that two groups are not different.

As previously noted, researchers often formulate a second, alternate version of their hypothesis called the research hypothesis (Patten, 2007). The alternate or research hypothesis is usually stated in a positive form.

Table 3–2. Examples of null hypotheses (H_0) and research hypotheses (H_1) for relational and difference studies

---

Relational study:

H_0: There is *no* relationship between CV ratio and mean length of utterance in preschool children from ages 18 to 36 months.

H_1: There is a significant relationship between CV ratio and mean length of utterance in preschool children from ages 18 to 36 months.

Difference study—nonexperimental:

H_0: CV ratio will *not* be different in 24-month-old children with normal hearing compared to 24-month-old children with moderate-to-severe hearing loss.

H_1: CV ratio will be different in 24-month-old children with normal hearing compared to 24-month-old children with moderate-to-severe hearing loss.

Difference study—experimental:

H_0: CV ratios for 24-month-old children with expressive language delay who participated in an 8-week intervention program will *not* be different from the CV ratios of 24-month-old children with expressive language delay who received no intervention.

H_1: CV ratios for 24-month-old children with expressive language delay who participated in an 8-week intervention program will be different from the CV ratios of 24-month-old children with expressive language delay who received no intervention.

The research hypothesis is a statement of what the researchers expected to find when they conducted their study. For example, theoretical models and previous research with other populations might all support the prediction that two variables are closely related. When researchers study these two variables in a new population, they expect the variable to be closely related when measured in the new population as well. This expectation is reflected in their statement of a research hypothesis. Table 3–2 includes examples of the alternate or research hypothesis that corresponds to each of the null hypotheses.

The research hypothesis might be stated as a *directional* hypothesis or as a *nondirectional* hypothesis (Patten, 2007). Each of the example research hypotheses in Table 3–2 was a nondirectional hypothesis. Although the researchers stated that they expected to find significant relationships between two variables or a significant difference between two groups, they did not indicate whether the relationship would be positive or negative, or which group would achieve higher scores. If researchers had reason to expect a particular outcome, such as a positive relationship between two variables or significantly higher scores for children in a treatment group, the researchers could formulate directional research hypotheses. In the examples in Table 3–3, each of the nondirectional research hypotheses

Table 3–3. Examples of nondirectional and directional research hypotheses (H_1) for relational and difference studies

---

Relational study:

Nondirectional H_1: There is a significant relationship between CV ratio and mean length of utterance in preschool children from ages 18 to 36 months.

Directional H_1: There is a significant *positive* relationship between CV ratio and mean length of utterance in preschool children from ages 18 to 36 months.

Difference study—nonexperimental:

Nondirectional H_1: CV ratio will be different in 24-month-old children with normal hearing compared to 24-month-old children with moderate-to-severe hearing loss.

Directional H_1: CV ratio will be *higher* in 24-month-old children with normal hearing compared to 24-month-old children with moderate-to-severe hearing loss.

Difference study—experimental:

Nondirectional H_1: CV ratios for 24-month-old children with expressive language delay who participated in an 8-week intervention program will be different from the CV ratios of 24-month-old children with expressive language delay who received no intervention.

Directional H_1: CV ratios for 24-month-old children with expressive language delay who participated in an 8-week intervention program will be *higher than* the CV ratios of 24-month-old children with expressive language delay who received no intervention.

---

from Table 3–2 is paired with a corresponding directional version.

Although the research and null hypotheses are a traditional way of defining the problem in quantitative studies, most authors of recent research articles choose other ways to state their problem. A perusal of articles published in the field of communication sciences and disorders in the last 5 years revealed that most articles include either research questions or a statement of purpose. However, the differences among research hypotheses, research questions, and statements of purpose are more differences in the form of the statement than differences in the content. Often a research question or statement of purpose includes the same information one would find in a research hypothesis.

Let's consider the following hypothetical study. A group of researchers developed a measure for assessing the intelligibility of conversational speech. They felt their new approach would be less time consuming and just as accurate as several existing measures of speech intelligibility. However, they needed to conduct a study to determine if these assumptions about their new measure were true. We will call the new measure the *conversational speech intelligibility index* or CSII. The researchers decided to conduct a study to compare scores on their CSII to scores on an existing speech intelligibility test. They expected to find a strong relationship between CSII performance and performance on the speech intelligibility test. Thus, they formulated the following research hypothesis:

H_1: There is a significant relationship between scores on the conversational speech intelligibility index and scores on an existing speech intelligibility test in children between the ages of 3 and 5 who have been diagnosed with a phonological disorder.

However, the researchers could just as easily have stated the same information in the form of a research question. With some minor rewording you could develop a question such as the following:

1. Is there a significant relationship between scores on the conversational speech intelligibility index and scores on an existing speech intelligibility test in children between the ages of 3 and 5 who have been diagnosed with a phonological disorder?

Many research reports include yes/no questions similar to the above example. Nevertheless, some authors such as Patten (2007) have suggested that researchers should avoid using yes/no questions because they yield relatively uninteresting, discrete answers. Revising a yes/no question to generate a question starting with *what, how,* and so forth is relatively easy. For example, the question above could be restated as a what question:

2. What is the relationship between scores on the conversational speech intelligibility index and scores on an existing speech intelligibility test in children between the ages of 3 and 5 who have been diagnosed with a phonological disorder?

According to Patten (2007), stating a research question as a what or a how question allows a researcher to give an answer that is less discrete and more elaborate. For example, in answering the what version of our example research question, a researcher could discuss the existence of a relationship between the measures, the direction of any relationship (e.g., positive or negative), as well as the strength of the relationship. Given a lack of consistent guidance regarding how to formulate research questions, deciding whether to use a yes/no version or a what/how version is largely a matter of personal preference.

Researchers also have the option of presenting the problem they intend to investigate in a *statement of purpose*. Like research questions, a statement of purpose usually includes the same kinds of information one would find in a formal hypothesis. However, a statement of purpose is a highly flexible form, not tied closely to quantitative research and statistical analysis. A statement of purpose would be an appropriate way to explain the focus on nearly any type of research including descriptive, relational, and difference studies. Using our previous example, we could generate a very similar statement of purpose for our hypothetical study. Such a statement might read as follows:

The purpose of this study was to investigate the relationship between a new measure of speech intelligibility, the conversational speech intelligibility index, and an existing speech intelligibility test when used with children between the ages of 3 and 5 who have been diagnosed with a phonological disorder.

When you begin reading research reports on a regular basis, you will occasionally encounter an additional approach to the problem statement, a *conditional* or *if-then* statement. When a study has theoretical implications, researchers sometimes prefer to state the problem in a conditional format. The general basis of conditional statements is that if the findings turn out one way, the study supports a certain conclusion; but if the findings turn out another way, the study supports a different conclusion. In a recent study, Coady, Evans, Mainela-Arnold, and Kluender (2007) used conditional statements to express possible outcomes for their study of speech perception in children with specific language impairment (SLI). The following examples of if-then statements are from Coady et al. (2007, p. 43).

If children with SLI are sensitive to speech quality, then they should perceive synthetic speech series less categorically than naturally spoken series. If they are sensitive to the lexical status of test items, then they should perceive nonsense-syllable test series less categorically than real-word test series. If their performance suffers from both of these manipulations, then only their perception of naturally spoken real words should match that of age-matched control children.

As noted in Chapter 1, authors usually explain the focus of their study in a paragraph that immediately precedes the results section of a research report. Thus, when you read an article, look for the research hypotheses, questions, or statement of purpose right before the methods section. When you read these questions or statements, you might find it helpful to look for information about how the outcomes were measured, that is, the dependent variables, and if appropriate, what variables the authors compared or manipulated (the independent variables).

Evidence-Based Practice Questions

In the previous section we covered the kinds of research questions and statements that guide empirical research. Empirical research involves gathering new information to answer questions that are important in the field of communication sciences and disorders. However, another kind of research question, an *evidence-based practice ques-*

tion, is of critical importance to audiologists and speech-language pathologists who are providing clinical services. When clinicians ask an evidence-based practice (EBP) question, they generally expect to find an answer to their question in the existing, published research literature. Sometimes clinicians have questions about the evidence associated with a particular etiology (e.g., Casby, 2001), or the reliability and validity of an assessment procedure, but most often clinicians have questions about the effectiveness of treatment for a particular disorder (e.g., Andrews, Guitar, & Howie, 1980; Conture, 1996; Law, Garrett, & Nye, 2004; Millar, Light, & Schlosser, 2006; Robey, 1998).

Sometimes audiologists and speech-language pathologists have EBP questions that are general in nature. For example, they might need to document the effectiveness of a particular intervention approach to meet a requirement of their work setting or of a funding or regulatory agency; or they might need information about a particular etiology to answer questions from a client or a client's family. These broad questions might take a form such as:

1. What evidence is available to document the effectiveness of language intervention for children in elementary school?
2. What evidence is available to document the effectiveness of behavioral treatment for adults who stutter?
3. What evidence is available to document the relative effectiveness of digital hearing aids in comparison to analog hearing aids?

Questions similar to those posed above were addressed in published reviews of language intervention for school-age children (Cirrin & Gillam, 2008), treatment for persons who stutter (Bothe, Davidow, Bramlett, & Ingham, 2006), effectiveness of digital hearing aids compared to analog (Taylor, Paisley, & Davis, 2001), and treatment for persons with aphasia (Robey, 1998). Robey (1998) noted that clinicians also might be interested in more specific questions addressing how treatment effectiveness is influenced by factors such as the amount of treatment, the severity of the person's disorder, or the kind of disorder.

Another way that audiologists and speech-language pathologists might approach EBP is to ask client-specific questions (Gallagher, 2002). When looking for evidence on behalf of an individual client, the clinician formulates a question that includes information about the client's disorder, his or her age, and the severity of the disorder (Gallagher, 2002). If clinicians have a question about intervention, they might include information about the specific form of treatment, the amount and/or frequency of treatment, and perhaps the expected amount of improvement (Gallagher, 2002). Each of the following example questions illustrates the features of a client-specific, treatment-specific question.

1. Will minimal pair phonological treatment, provided for two 30-minute individual treatment sessions per week for 16 weeks, produce a 20% gain in percentage of consonants correct in spontaneous speech for a 5-year-old child with a moderately severe speech production disorder?

2. Will early detection of hearing loss and amplification fitting prior to 6 months of age result in age-appropriate scores on a test of expressive and receptive language at age 2 for a child with a severe hearing loss, when provided without additional speech and language intervention?

The client-specific EBP question is the starting point for a literature search rather than for original, empirical research. In searching the literature, the clinician will focus on those studies that more closely match the client and treatment characteristics specified in the question. For question 1 above, the clinician would look for studies that addressed minimal pair phonological treatment, included participants who were approximately 5 years of age, and ideally had moderate-to-severe speech production disorders. For question 2, the clinician would look for studies of early detection and treatment of children with severe hearing loss that included long-term follow-up and assessment of the children's speech and language development at approximately age 2. When audiologists and speech-language pathologists search for research evidence on behalf of an individual client, they need to keep in mind that they might not find studies that perfectly fit the criteria of their question. In such instances, clinicians need to decide if studies that meet only some of their criteria are useful. For example, they need to consider whether or not research conducted with participants who were a different age, had less severe disorders, or had different language backgrounds is useful for guiding their clinical decisions.

Criteria for
Well-Formed Questions

Whether your intent is to conduct an empirical study or to conduct an EBP search of the literature, an important step in the early phase of your research is to generate a well-formed question. One consideration in writing a research question is to include sufficient detail in the descriptions of your variables. Additionally, the experimental treatment needs to be one that other audiologists and speech-language pathologists could carry out in a similar way (i.e., reliable procedure). The term *operationalize* refers to a process in which researchers provide a precise, specific description of the independent and dependent variables in their study. An independent variable could be described in terms of the procedures associated with an experimental treatment, whereas a dependent variable could be defined in terms of a specific measure or test. Although a well-written research question should include specific information, a researcher might only partially define the variables in the questions or statement of purpose and provide a full description in the methods section of a research report. Table 3–4 includes a set of statements illustrating the difference between general and specific descriptions of both independent and dependent variables.

Another characteristic of a well-written research question is that the variables are defined in a way that leads to valid and reliable conclusions.[2] When choosing ways to measure outcomes, researchers should consider the validity and reliability of the measures. The *validity* of a measurement refers to how accurately a test or measure represents the knowledge, skill, or trait you set out to assess. Further, an instrument has an intended purpose and conclusions about validity are based on the extent to which it accomplishes that purpose (Patten, 2007).

The *reliability* of a measure refers to the extent to which the measure yields con-

---

[2]Usually we apply the concepts of validity and reliability to dependent variables or outcome measurements. Trochim and Donnelly (2007) noted that independent variables also should be implemented in a way that supports the validity and reliability of conclusions regarding experimental manipulations. For example, a researcher testing a new treatment approach needs to plan a treatment that others in the field would recognize as a valuable one (i.e., valid treatment).

Table 3–4. Statements illustrating the difference between general and specific descriptions of research variables

General Statement	Specific Statement
1. Children with language disorders	1. Children who scored more than 1.5 standard deviations below the mean on the Test of Language Development–Primary, 3rd edition
2. Adults with aphasia	2. Adults who received a score of 90 or less on the Aphasia Quotient of the Western Aphasia Battery
3. Children with bilateral hearing loss	3. Children with an average pure-tone threshold above 50 dB bilaterally
4. Phonological treatment	4. Hodson's cycles phonological treatment approach
5. Treatment for voice disorders	5. Sixteen ½-hour sessions of resonance voice therapy over 8 weeks
6. Improved speech production	6. Higher percentage of intelligible words in a 200-word conversational speech sample
7. Improved speech perception	7. Higher scores on the revised Speech Perception in Noise test

sistent or repeatable results (Rosenthal & Rosnow, 2008). When judging reliability, one might consider consistency of measurement from one time to another, from one person to another, from one form of a test to another, or from one subset of test items to another. The different ways of establishing reliability and validity will be discussed in the following section. A statement frequently associated with the concepts of reliability and validity is that a measure can be reliable even if it is not valid, but a measure cannot be valid if it is not reliable (Patten, 2007).[3] The most preferred measures are those that have both high validity and high reliability (Rosenthal & Rosnow, 2008).

Establishing Validity and Reliability

One way to show that findings of a study are accurate and meaningful is to choose measurement procedures or tests that have known validity and reliability. Most published tests in audiology and speech-language pathology include information in their test manuals about both validity and reliability. However, on occasion the most appropriate outcome measures for a study might be novel or unpublished procedures. In these situations researchers usually include information in the methods section of the research

---

[3]Although generally accepted as true, this statement may have some exceptions. Rosenthal and Rosnow (2008) described a rare situation in which a measure could be valid even though it was not reliable.

report about how they established the reliability of the measurements.

Professionals who are developing a test for publication or trying to document the appropriateness of a measurement approach for an empirical study have a number of choices regarding how to demonstrate the validity and reliability of their procedures. We cover the most common approaches to establishing validity and reliability in this section. For validity, these approaches include face validity, criterion validity, content validity, and construct validity. For reliability, these approaches include interobserver reliability, test-retest reliability, parallel forms reliability, and internal consistency reliability. As we discuss these various approaches, keep in mind that a test or procedure is valid for a specific purpose and reliable under certain circumstances. For example, a test of vocabulary comprehension would be appropriate for some situations, but not if you are trying to assess higher-order language use such as drawing inferences or recognizing word relationships. Similarly, a test might be a reliable measure when the client is attentive and focused on the task, but not when the client is inattentive or focused on some extraneous environmental stimulus. Further, decisions about the validity or reliability of a test are not dichotomous (e.g., a valid or invalid test; a reliable or unreliable test). Rather, these decisions reflect the degree to which a test is valid or the degree to which it is reliable.

Professionals in various fields have ideas about the areas they usually assess or measure. A person who is reasonably well trained in the content of their field should have an informed opinion regarding what should be measured to document abilities such as language comprehension, speech sound production, speech recognition, and so forth. We use the term *face validity* to refer to validity based on a person's judg-

ment of how well a test appears to accomplish its purpose. When professionals in communication sciences and disorders examine a test or other instrument and decide that it appears to have appropriate content we could say that the test has face validity. Face validity might be regarded as a rather informal approach to establishing validity because it is based on individual ideas regarding appropriate content or procedures. Persons examining a test use their own internal standards when judging face validity rather than some type of empirical evidence. In some applications of face validity the judges are untrained persons rather than professionals such as audiologists or speech-language pathologists. The notion of obtaining the opinions of untrained persons makes sense when you consider that the persons who take speech, language, or hearing tests usually are not trained in the fields of audiology or speech-language pathology. The persons who take tests might be more likely to maintain high motivation and attention to the task if they perceive that the test they are taking is an appropriate and meaningful way to assess their knowledge or skills. In a way face validity might be thought of as the validity established by consumers. The consumers for speech, language, and hearing tests are the audiologists and speech-language pathologists who purchase the tests and their clients who take the tests.

The term *content validity* refers to another way of establishing validity using judgment. However, demonstrating the content validity of a test usually involves a comparatively formal approach. Rosenthal and Rosnow (2008, p. 113) noted that a test with good content validity includes the " . . . kinds of material (or content areas) . . . " an expert in the field would expect. Another aspect of content validity is that authors base their testing approach on a model or theory that is well known. For example, tests of language abilities generally address components of language such as syntax, morphology, and semantics. Tests of word recognition usually include words that represent the phonological system of the target language. Often, test authors recruit a panel of experts to review a test before publishing it. These experts carefully examine the test and judge its content. They base their judgments on how well the test represents the underlying model or theory and how broadly it samples the expected content. The judges may also consider whether or not the test employs appropriate response modes, provides material in a motivating and attractive format, and addresses different skill levels such as recalling basic facts and definitions or drawing inferences. A test author in the field of communication sciences and disorders would recruit a panel of judges who are highly respected in the field of audiology or speech-language pathology. These individuals will draw on their knowledge of the field of audiology or speech-language pathology, on the information the test authors provide about the theory underlying the test, and also on their knowledge of the characteristics of better-quality tests. Often test authors revise the original version of a test based on the feedback they receive from this panel of experts. For example, they might eliminate, reword, or add some test items.

A third way to determine test validity is *criterion validity*. This is an empirical approach to validity that involves comparing a new test or measure to an existing one that serves as the standard of comparison (Patten, 2007). One way to establish criterion validity is to recruit a group of participants and administer both the new test and the standard, comparison test to these participants. When you administer the new test and the criterion measure relatively close

together, you are establishing the *concurrent validity* of your test. That is, you determine that the new test measures a content area in a way that is similar to the existing test, when the participants take the tests at approximately the same time.

Another form of criterion validity is when you administer the new test to a group of participants and determine how they perform on a criterion measure in the future. This latter type of criterion validity is sometimes called *predictive validity*. When scores on a test are valuable for predicting success in a future activity, such as career success, graduate school performance, or reading achievement, the test is said to have predictive validity. To establish predictive validity, test developers conduct a longitudinal study in which they administer their new assessment approach to a group of participants and then follow those participants over time, often a year or more later. The participants are reevaluated at the later time to determine if scores on the new test successfully predicted their future performance. An example of predictive validity is when educators or speech-language pathologists administered phoneme awareness tasks to children at approximately age 4 or 5 to determine if phonemic awareness abilities predicted future reading achievement. When the children were older, perhaps in first or second grade, the researchers assessed their reading skills and compared their reading scores to their earlier scores on the phonemic awareness tasks.

One might wonder about the logic of comparing a new test to one that serves as a standard of comparison. If a test is available that audiologists or speech-language pathologists regard as the standard way of assessing a particular communication behavior, why would you need to develop a new test? Authors might have several reasons for developing a new assessment procedure.

One reason could be to develop a shorter version of a test that takes less time to administer. A "short form" of an assessment might be published as a standalone test or as a subtest within a comprehensive assessment tool. An example of this would be when authors of a language test include a subtest to assess vocabulary comprehension. In this situation test authors might compare their new subtest to the Peabody Picture Vocabulary Test–III, which could serve as the standard of comparison for vocabulary comprehension tests. Another example of this is when audiologists explored the use of shorter word lists to assess word recognition abilities of persons with hearing loss (Runge & Hosford-Dunn, 1985). In this case, the researchers compared their participants' performance on the short form of the test with the full test to determine if the two versions yielded similar results. Other reasons to develop a new test procedure and compare it to an existing test are when test authors believe the existing test has weaknesses that they have eliminated in their new test, or when test authors are developing a series of tests that assess various aspects of speech, language, or hearing.

When authors want to compare scores on a new test they are developing to scores on an existing standard of comparison they might choose to compute a *validity coefficient*. A validity coefficient is similar to a correlation coefficient and ranges from 0.0 to 1.00. If a new test has no relationship to the standard of comparison, the validity coefficient will be low (e.g., approaching 0.0), but if the new test has a strong relationship to the standard of comparison the validity coefficient will be high (e.g., approaching 1.0). Ideally, test developers want to obtain relatively high coefficients when they compute validity coefficients. Guidelines for interpreting correlation coefficients suggest that a correlation of approx-imately 0.75 or higher would be a strong correlation (Patten, 2007); similarly, a validity coefficient of 0.75 or higher would indicate a strong relationship between new and comparison tests. Patten (2007) noted that even somewhat lower coefficients would be acceptable in some situations. This would be true when examining predictors of activities or achievements that have multiple influences, such as performance at work or school achievement. A single predictor measure such as a test of discipline-specific knowledge would only capture some of the influences on future job performance. Another caution to keep in mind is that a strong validity coefficient only has value if test developers have confidence that the standard of comparison was itself a valid assessment tool. For example, if the goal was to develop a measure that would predict future success as an audiologist or speech-language pathologist, the standard of comparison probably should be some measure of future performance in a clinical setting. Grades in graduate level courses would not be a meaningful standard of comparison when the goal is to predict clinical skill.

Construct validity, the final method for establishing validity, might be the most challenging to understand. As noted earlier, test developers often design a test to fit a particular theory or model. The theory or model provides guidance regarding what behaviors to sample and how to design questions to test those behaviors. One application of a theory is to develop a series of constructs that a test is intended to measure. Patten (2007, p. 69) explained a construct as " . . . a collection of related behaviors that are associated in a meaningful way." Thus, test developers might design a test with a set of questions to sample one or more behavioral constructs. To establish construct validity, test developers analyze patterns of performance on test items to determine if they reflect the underlying theory or model. This theory or model is manifested in the behavioral constructs the test samples.

One way to establish construct validity is to look at patterns or relationships among test items, or relationships between test items and external standards of comparison. One kind of relationship that provides support for a behavioral construct is *convergence* (Rosenthal & Rosnow, 2008). When a person performs in a similar way on test items the items might be said to exhibit convergence. Similarly, when a person performs in a similar way on two different tests that appear to test the same content, the two tests might be said to exhibit convergence. Another kind of relationship that is important for establishing the validity of a behavioral construct is a *divergent* relationship. A divergent relationship might emerge when a researcher compares a person's performance on test items that represent two different behavioral constructs. For example, a test might include items that assess an individual's motor skills and other items that assess cognitive abilities. A person could have very good cognitive abilities and relatively poorer motor skills, and thus, scores from items that tap cognitive abilities could be quite different from scores on items that tap motor skills. A meaningful behavioral construct, as represented by performance on a set of test items, should exhibit both patterns of convergence and divergence, and analyzing patterns of convergent and divergent relationships among test items is one way to establish construct validity.

Let's consider an example from the field of speech-language pathology. Oral language is a content that speech-language pathologists frequently assess. A hypothetical model of oral language skills might include language components such as phonology, syntax, morphology and semantics, as well as expressive and receptive language skills.

The behavioral constructs for such a model might be areas such as syntax in expressive language and receptive language, semantics in expressive language and receptive language, and so forth. When conducting a study to analyze how well a test samples these constructs, a researcher would expect to find the closest relationships among test items that sample the same behavioral construct. Thus, a strong relationship or convergence should emerge among items that sample syntax in expressive language, but these items should show a weak relationship or divergence when compared to items that sample a different behavioral construct such as semantics in receptive language. Similarly, if researchers compared performance on the new test items to performance on an external standard, they would expect to find convergence when the two tests sample similar behavioral constructs (e.g., a subtest that samples expressive morphology compared to an established test of expressive morphology) but divergence when the two tests sample different behavioral constructs (e.g., the subtest that samples expressive morphology compared to an established test of receptive vocabulary).

Like the options available for establishing validity, researchers and test developers also have several options for determining the reliability of their assessment procedures. Remember that reliability refers to the extent to which a test yields consistent results (Patten, 2007; Rosenthal & Rosnow, 2008). For the purposes of discussion, our focus will be on four of the ways of establishing reliability: interobserver reliability, test-retest reliability, parallel forms reliability, and split-half reliability.

If a measurement procedure has *interobserver reliability*, the procedure is one that yields consistent results when two different examiners or observers use the procedure to test the same persons. To establish interobserver reliability, researchers and test developers usually recruit a group of participants, and then ask different examiners to test these participants using the same test procedures. The participants are tested twice, usually at about the same time (such as both test administrations within 2 weeks of each other). With two scores for each participant, you can compute a correlation coefficient to determine the degree of reliability. A strong correlation means that the different examiners obtained similar results. Persons who scored high when tested by the first examiner also scored high when tested by the second examiner; conversely, persons who scored low when tested by the first examiner also scored low when tested by the second examiner.

To establish *test-retest reliability*, the researchers once again recruit a group of participants and test them at two different times. However, with test-retest reliability the same examiner usually administers both tests. If a measurement procedure has strong test-retest reliability, the measure yields consistent results from one time to the next when administered by the same person. As with interobserver reliability, you can compute a correlation coefficient to determine the degree of test-retest reliability once you obtain two scores for each participant. Selecting a measure with strong test-retest reliability is an important consideration when conducting a study of treatment outcomes, because you need a measure that yields stable results from one test administration to the next. That way, it is more likely that the changes you observe from the beginning to end of the study relate to the treatment received and not to measurement instability.

In *parallel-forms reliability*, the researchers or test developers construct two different, but hopefully equivalent, forms of a measure. The two forms include comparable test items and measure the same behavioral construct(s). Researchers conduct a study similar to the ones described above to determine if two different versions of a measure have parallel-forms reliability. However, in this case they administer one form to the participants first, and then administer the second form a short time later. Again, because you have two scores from each participant, you can compute a correlation coefficient to determine the degree of reliability between the two parallel forms.

A final type of reliability is *split-half reliability*. To determine this type of reliability, you administer a test once to your participants. Following test administration, you split the test items into two equivalent forms and then compare the participants' scores for each form. One common way to divide a test into equivalent halves is to split it into odd-numbered and even-numbered items. Rosenthal and Rosnow (2008) noted that obtaining two equivalent forms can be problematic depending on how the test is constructed and how it is divided. Generally, a measure that samples a single behavioral construct with a set of similar items would be easier to divide into equal halves than a measure that samples several behavioral constructs with different types of items. Because you obtain two scores from each participant, you can compute a correlation coefficient between the two halves of the test. However, this correlation might underrepresent the actual reliability of the entire test because reliability is influenced by the number of items on a test (Trochim & Donnelly, 2007).[4] Split-half reliability is regarded as a measure of internal consistency (Trochim & Donnelly, 2007). That

---

[4]Trochim and Donnelly (2007) identified a more accurate approach, the Spearman-Brown formula, for estimating the reliability of an entire test based on the split-half correlation. Discussion of this approach is beyond the scope of this text.

is, the correlation between two halves of a test reflects the extent to which items on the test measure the same behavioral construct. Although the split-half reliability procedure has some limitations, one advantage is that you can determine this type of reliability from a single test administration. This could be an advantage for a researcher who wants to establish the reliability and internal consistency of a novel assessment procedure.

As noted previously, determining reliability of an assessment procedure is a matter of degree. Computing correlation coefficients for interobserver, test-retest, or other forms of reliability provides quantitative information about the level of reliability. The level of reliability you need depends on how you plan to use the scores. Audiologists and speech-language pathologists who are testing individual clients and making decisions based on the client's test scores need measures with high reliability. Higher reliabilities are necessary when individual scores will be interpreted. However, if you are going to base your conclusions on mean group scores, somewhat lower reliability coefficients are tolerable. This would be the case for a researcher who has tested many participants with the intention of comparing the scores of different groups.

conducting a literature search. Regardless of the nature of the research, whether it is a descriptive, relational, or difference study, or whether it is an evidence-based practice search, researchers will be more successful if they develop a well-formed research question. In writing their questions, researchers consider ways to describe their manipulations or independent variables and outcome or dependent variables in a precise and specific way. The term *operationalize* refers to this process of defining the variables in a study. Researchers also need to establish that the information they obtain is both valid and reliable. Validity refers to how accurately a measure or procedure represents an actual behavioral construct. Reliability refers to the extent to which a measure or procedure yields consistent or repeatable results. The options for establishing validity of a measure include face, criterion, content, and construct validity. Face validity could be established in a relatively informal way, but researchers and test developers conduct specific kinds of studies to establish the other forms of validity. Researchers also have several options for establishing reliability, including interobserver reliability, test-retest reliability, parallel forms reliability, and internal consistency reliability. The best measures and procedures for answering researchers' questions are those that have both high validity and reliability.

Summary

The starting point for most research is a question or problem a researcher or clinician wants to explore. Usually these unanswered questions emerge from our reading of professional literature or from the problems clients present when we provide audiology and speech-language pathology services. A well-written research question provides guidance for designing original research or

Review Questions

H_0: Children who participate in the dynamic intervention approach will not have different intelligibility scores and accuracy of sound production in conversational speech after 12 weeks of treatment than children who participate in the traditional articulation approach.

H_1: Children who participate in the dynamic intervention approach will have higher intelligibility scores and accuracy of sound production in conversational speech after 12 weeks of treatment than children who participate in the traditional articulation approach.

1. The statement labeled H_0 above is called a _____, and the statement labeled H_1 is called a _____.

2. In either H_0 or H_1 above, what is the independent variable? The dependent variable?

3. Is H_1 in the example directional or nondirectional? If it is directional, rewrite it to be nondirectional. If it is nondirectional, rewrite it to be directional.

4. Another approach to defining the focus of a study is to write a research question. Rewrite H_1 above as a research question.

5. How might an author of a research paper include the information in these examples in a statement of purpose? Write an example.

6. Consider the dependent variable(s) in H_0 or H_1. How might you *operationalize* the dependent variable(s) to make them more measurable?

7. Think of an area of communication sciences and disorders that interests you. What are some of the measurement instruments used in this area? What do you know about their reliability and validity?

8. What type of reliability is important for measuring the outcomes of a treatment study? How do you establish this type of reliability?

9. Try to identify an area in communication sciences and disorders for which you would want to make predictions. How could you establish the predictive validity of a measure for this purpose?

10. A validity coefficient is based on what statistic? Given the nature of this statistic, a validity coefficient would range from _____ to _____.

11. If a test yields consistent results, it is a _____ test.

12. Identify the most accurate statement:
    a. A speech, language, or hearing test with high reliability might have low validity.
    b. A speech, language, or hearing test with high validity might have low reliability.

13. Describe each of the following forms of reliability:
    a. Interobserver reliability
    b. Test-retest reliability
    c. Parallel-forms reliability
    d. Split-half reliability

14. Which statement is true?
    a. We test our subjects at two different times to establish split-half reliability.
    b. We test our subjects at two different times to establish test-retest reliability.

Learning Activities

1. Read the introductory section of one or more of the following research articles. These articles illustrate different ways of defining the focus of a study such as using hypotheses, research questions, or a statement of purpose.

Hypotheses

Lane, H., Denny, M., Guenther, F. H., Hanson, H. M., Marrone, N., Mathies, M. L., et al. (2007). On the structure of phoneme categories in listeners with cochlear implants. *Journal of Speech-Language-Hearing Research, 50,* 2-14.

Yes/No Questions

Pfyler, P. N., Lowery, K. J., Hamby, H. M., & Trine, T. D. (2007). The objective and subjective evaluation of multichannel expansion in wide dynamic range compression hearing instruments. *Journal of Speech-Language-Hearing Research, 50,* 15-24.

If-Then Statements

Coady, J. A., Evans, J. L., Mainela-Arnold, E., & Kluender, K. R. (2007). Children with specific language impairments perceive speech most categorically when tokens are natural and meaningful. *Journal of Speech-Language-Hearing Research, 50,* 41-57.

Statements of Purpose

Stierwalt, J. A. G., & Youmans, S. R. (2007). Tongue measures in individuals with normal and impaired swallowing. *American Journal of Speech-Language Pathology, 16,* 148-156.

Zekveld, A. A., Deijen, J. B., Goverts, S. T., & Kramer, S. E. (2007). The relationship between nonverbal cognitive functions and hearing loss. *Journal of Speech-Language-Hearing Research, 50,* 74-82.

2. Read the manual for one or more of the following speech and language tests or other tests of your choosing. Look for information about how the authors established the reliability and validity of their tests.

Boehm, A. E. (2001). *Boehm test of basic concepts: Examiner's manual* (3rd ed.). San Antonio, TX: The Psychological Corporation.

Dabul, B. L. (2000). *Apraxia battery for adults: Examiner's manual* (2nd ed.). Austin, TX: Pro-ed.

Dunn, L. M., Dunn, D. M. (2007). *Peabody picture vocabulary test: Manual* (4th ed.). San Antonio, TX: Harcourt Assessment.

Hodson, B. W., (2004). *Hodson assessment of phonological patterns: Examiner's manual.* (3rd ed.). Austin, TX: Pro-ed.

Kertesz, A. (2006). *Western aphasia battery—revised: Examiner's Manual.* San Antonio, TX: Harcourt Assessment.

Lippke, B. A., Dickey, S. E., Selman, J. W., & Soder, A. L. (1997). *Photo articulation test: Examiner's manual* (3rd ed.). Austin, TX: Pro-ed.

Zimmerman, I. L., Steiner, V. G., & Pond, R. E. (2002). *Preschool language scale: Examiner's manual* (4th ed.). an Antonio, TX: The Psychological Corporation.

References

American Speech-Language-Hearing Association. (2004). *Evidence-based practice in communication disorders: An introduction* [Technical report]. Retrieved January 3, 2007, from http://www.asha.org/docs/html/TR2004-00001.html

Andrews, G., Guitar, B., & Howie, P. (1980). Meta-analysis of the effects of stuttering treatment.

Journal of Speech and Hearing Disorders, 45, 287–307.

Barnett, W. S. (2000). Economics of early childhood intervention. In J. P. Shonkoff & S. J. Meisels (Eds.), *Handbook of early childhood intervention* (2nd ed., pp. 589–610). Cambridge, UK: Cambridge University Press.

Bothe, A. K., Davidow, J. H., Bramlett, R. E., & Ingham, R. J. (2006). Stuttering treatment research 1970–2005: I. Systematic review incorporating trial quality assessment of behavioral, cognitive, and related approaches. *American Journal of Speech-Language Pathology, 15*, 321–341.

Casby, M. W. (2001). Otitis media and language development: A meta-analysis. *American Journal of Speech-Language Pathology, 10*, 65–80.

Cirrin, F. M., & Gillam, R. B. (2008). Language intervention practices for school-age children with spoken language disorders: A systematic review. *Language, Speech, and Hearing Services in Schools, 39*, S110–S137.

Coady, J. A., Evans, J. L., Mainela-Arnold, E., & Kluender, K. R. (2007). Children with specific language impairments perceive speech most categorically when tokens are natural and meaningful. *Journal of Speech-Language-Hearing Research, 50*, 41–57.

Conture, E. G. (1996). Treatment efficacy: Stuttering. *Journal of Speech and Hearing Research, 39*, S18–S26.

Foster, S. L., & Mash, E. J. (1999). Assessing social validity in clinical treatment research: Issues and procedures [Electronic version]. *Journal of Consulting and Clinical Psychology, 67*(3), 308–319.

Gallagher, T. M. (2002). Evidence-based practice: Applications to speech-language pathology. *Perspectives on Language Learning and Education, 9*(1), 2–5.

Law, J., Garrett, Z., & Nye, C. (2004). The efficacy of treatment for children with developmental speech and language delay/disorder: A meta-analysis. *Journal of Speech, Language, and Hearing Research, 47*, 924–943.

Millar, D. C., Light, J. C., & Schlosser, R. W. (2006). The impact of augmentative and alternative communication intervention on the speech production of individuals with developmental disabilities: A research review. *Journal of Speech, Language, and Hearing Research, 49*, 248–264.

Patten, M. L. (2007). *Understanding research methods: An overview of the essentials* (6th ed.). Glendale, CA: Pyrczak.

Robey, R. R. (1998). A meta-analysis of clinical outcomes in the treatment of aphasia. *Journal of Speech-Language-Hearing Research, 41*, 172–187.

Rosenthal, R., & Rosnow, R. L. (2008). *Essentials of behavioral research: Methods and data analysis* (3rd ed.). New York: McGraw Hill.

Runge, C. A., & Hosford-Dunn, H. (1985). Word recognition performance with modified CID W-22 word lists. *Journal of Speech and Hearing Research, 28*, 355–362.

Silverman, F. H. (1998). *Research design and evaluation in speech-language pathology and audiology: Asking and answering questions* (4th ed.). Englewood Cliffs, NJ: Prentice Hall.

Taylor, R. S., Paisley, S., & Davis, A. (2001). Systematic review of the clinical and cost effectiveness of digital hearing aids. *British Journal of Audiology, 35*(5), 271–288.

Trochim, W. M. K., & Donnelly, J. P. (2007). *The research methods knowledge base* (3rd ed.). Mason, OH: Thomson Custom.

CHAPTER 4

Completing a Literature Search

Audiologists and speech-language patholo-gists working in clinical settings, as well as researchers planning an original study, need to be skilled at finding, evaluating, and sum-marizing information. *Information literacy* is a term often used to refer to the skills associated with finding, evaluating, summa-rizing, and using information (American Library Association [ALA], 2006). For audi-ologists and speech-language pathologists, the emerging emphasis on evidence-based practice has made information literacy skills even more important. For researchers, information literacy skills have always been an essential part of finding problems to study and of defining and researching those problems in ways that yield valid and reli-able answers.

When professionals, such as those in communication sciences and disorders, medicine, or psychology, look for informa-tion, we usually conduct a *literature search*. The intent of a literature search is to find information within a body of written work that pertains to our topic. Audiologists and speech-language pathologists might search within the body of written work for com-munication sciences and disorders, or within the body of written work for related fields such as education, medicine, neuroscience,

or psychology. A successful literature search depends on information literacy skills such as knowing how to search, where to look, and how to define your topic. In the follow-ing sections of this chapter, we will cover the reasons for conducting a literature search, some general information about planning and conducting searches, and some begin-ning skills for reading, evaluating, and doc-umenting information. In the Appendix of this chapter we practice some sample searches to learn more about planning and conducting searches using some of the more readily available search tools. Some of you might skip this last section if you already feel comfortable with your ability to plan a search and find appropriate informa-tion on a topic.

Purposes of a Literature Search

Audiologists and speech-language patholo-gists have many reasons to conduct a litera-ture search. Sometimes the goal of the search is to *find an answer* to your question in the existing literature. This would be the case when conducting a search for evidence to answer clinical questions pertaining to the etiology, assessment, or treatment of communication disorders. In evidence-based practice (EBP) research, the aim is to find information that already exists in the body of written work in a particular field (Schardt & Mayer, 2004). Further, some of the published work in the field of communication sciences and disorders is nonempirical in nature. In empirical research the goal is to generate original evidence; however, in nonempirical research the goal is to identify all of the existing evidence on a particular topic. The author of a nonempirical work, such as a theoretical discussion or a systematic review, needs to conduct a thorough literature search in order to find all of the published work relevant to the topic. Even researchers who are planning an empirical study need to conduct a literature search to find out if their question has already been answered in an earlier study.

For those who are planning to conduct original, empirical research, finding that someone else conducted a study similar to the one you were planning does not necessarily mean you should abandon your idea. A field with a strong body of empirical research should have some studies that replicate the findings of earlier work. Sometimes the research in a field becomes outdated for reasons such as changes in population characteristics or the emergence of new tests or instruments to measure outcomes. Even for relatively recent studies, researchers could plan a study that replicates the results with slightly different procedures or participants (Patten, 2007).

Another reason for conducting a literature search is to find the *previous research on a topic*, even if that research does not answer your question directly. The previous research might be relevant even if it addressed a different population from the one you intended to study, looked at a different set of outcome measures, or even examined

a different approach to treatment. For example, researchers interested in studying the use of classroom amplification in college and university classrooms might find very little research in the college setting. However, they could include several studies of use of classroom amplification in elementary school classrooms in their review of literature. Researchers who designed a study of a particular approach to treatment, such as a treatment for persons with functional voice disorders, aphasia, or specific language impairment, usually would include information about other approaches to treatment in their review of prior research. In an EBP search, you might not find a study that exactly matched your client's age and severity of disorder or examined the treatment you wanted to investigate. However, the related research you do find might provide meaningful guidance for your clinical decisions.

Researchers who want to conduct an original, empirical study might conduct a literature search to *identify a problem* to study. The researchers might know the general topics in communication sciences and disorders they want to investigate but not have an idea for a specific research question. As we discussed in Chapter 3, sometimes the authors of a research report include specific suggestions for future studies in their discussion sections. Sometimes when you read a few articles on the same research topic, you find that the findings of the studies conflict. This is another way to find an interesting research question. You might consider any differences in the conflicting studies. For example, were the participants different in some way? Did one study include participants with more severe disorders or participants from different age groups? Or perhaps the researchers in one study administered their treatment for a longer time or measured their outcomes in different ways. Any differences you find could be good independent variables to investigate in a new study.

Perhaps you have an interest in another field of study in addition to communication sciences and disorders. You could find important questions to research by searching the literature to *identify methods from other fields of study*. If you looked at the reference lists for research articles in communication sciences and disorders, you might find citations from journals covering cognitive psychology, developmental psychology, neuroscience, psycholinguistics, and so forth. For example, a recent article on working memory in children with specific language impairment included citations from journals such as *Applied Psycholinguistics, Journal of Memory and Language, Memory and Cognition*, and *Psychological Review* (Marton & Schwartz, 2003); a 2007 report on elderly listeners' recognition of time-compressed speech included citations from the *Journal of the Acoustical Society of America, Journal of Gerontology, IEEE Transactions on Rehabilitation Engineering*, and *Psychology and Aging* (Gordon-Salant, Fitzgibbons, & Friedman, 2007).

Even when researchers know the research question they want to investigate, they might conduct a literature search to *generate background information* for use when writing their research report (Patten, 2007). This background information might include theories or models that pertain to the focus of the study, statistical information such as on the prevalence of a disorder, or definitions of important concepts. Finally, researchers might need to search the literature to *identify procedures or outcome measures* to use in their research. Possibly a researcher has a need to describe participants or document a treatment outcome in terms of the impact of the person's communication impairment on activity and participation in daily life (American Speech-Language-Hearing Association [ASHA], 2004; ASHA, 2006; Ma & Yiu, 2001; World Health Organization, 2001). This researcher could do a literature search to identify ways to document activity and participation restrictions. Other researchers might be interested in using a reaction time measurement in their study and might search the literature to determine how other researchers measured reaction times in their experiments.

A search of the existing research literature is an important early step in planning a study. Such a search might aid the researcher to find an interesting problem to study, to find new research approaches, or to find the background information they need to develop a strong justification for their research ideas. In the following section, we cover some of the tools a researcher could use to complete the important step of a literature search.

Planning and Conducting a Search

Search Tools

As you plan a literature search, one of the first considerations is how to find trustworthy, professional information in an efficient way. Generally, the most efficient way to find information is to use a *Web-based search engine*. You might already be familiar with very popular search engines such as *Google* (2007) or *Ask* (2008). These search engines provide a large amount of information on a topic in a short time. However, neither Google nor Ask would be an ideal choice when looking for literature in the field of communication sciences and disorders. When conducting an EBP search or planning scientific research, audiologists and speech-language pathologists need to search the evidence published in professional journals or presented at professional conferences. Usually, professional journals have procedures for peer review of submissions designed to ensure that published articles meet the journal's standards, are well written, and report on well-designed research. Although a Google or Ask search generally uncovers some professional literature, you also retrieve other kinds of information from commercial and even personal Web sites. Thus, when conducting a search for high quality information in communication sciences and disorders, you should use a search engine designed to retrieve peer-reviewed journal articles from various scientific disciplines.

Researchers have many search engines to employ when looking for professional literature. Covering all of the possible search engines is beyond the scope of this chapter; however, we will cover some of the most important search tools for audiologists and speech-language pathologists. Listed below are the search engines we will discuss.

1. Education Resources Information Center (ERIC)
2. PubMed
3. Professional association Web sites
4. Highwire Press
5. Google Scholar
6. ComDisDome via CSA Illumina
7. ScienceDirect
8. OhioLink
9. ProQuest

The on-line search engines listed above are not necessarily ordered according to which would be the best choice for a search. However, some of the search engines are provided without a fee and should be available to you throughout your professional career. Others are premium services that

might be available on many college and university campuses via site licenses.

The first two on-line search tools we will cover are databases provided by the U.S. government. The *ERIC database* is a research tool provided by the Institute of Education Sciences (IES; n.d.) and the U.S. Department of Education. ERIC provides a way to search approximately 600 journals in the field of education, including articles from journals in communication sciences and disorders (IES, n.d.). Although researchers usually use several on-line search engines, ERIC could be the primary search tool for research focusing on education, preschool and school-age children, language and literacy, and so forth. An ERIC search yields citation information such as author(s), title, journal, and usually an abstract of the article. Some articles in the ERIC database are available in full text form. The ERIC Web site provides both basic and advanced search strategies. The Appendix includes a description of a search using the ERIC advanced search option for those who would like specific information about using this tool.

PubMed is a Web-based tool for searching the Medline database, a major database of journal articles in medicine and other life science disciplines (National Center for Biotechnology Information [NCBI], 2007). PubMed is provided as a service of the National Library of Medicine and the U.S. National Institutes of Health. Like an ERIC search, a literature search with PubMed yields information such as the author(s), title, journal, and usually an abstract of the article. If a journal publisher has a Web site with full text versions of articles, a PubMed search also returns a link to that Web site. PubMed could be your primary search tool when looking for information on medical audiology or speech-language pathology; speech, language, or hearing disorders with an anatomical or physiological basis; and adult onset disorders such as sensorineural hearing loss, aphasia, and voice disorders. The PubMed search engine provides some helpful search tools such as the ability to set limits on publication dates, language, age groups, as well as type of article; and the process of *automatic term matching* provides matches on semantically similar terms (e.g., treatment, intervention, therapy) and grammatical variations (e.g., stutter, stuttering, stutters) (NCBI, 2007). The Appendix includes a description of a PubMed search where some of these tools are illustrated.

Professional associations such as the American Academy of Audiology (AAA), American Speech-Language-Hearing Association (ASHA), and American Psychological Association (APA) publish professional journals as a service to their members. One way to find articles in these journals is to search the association Web site. Usually even non-members are able to conduct a search of an association Web site, but they might not be able to view full text versions of the articles they retrieve. Members of the association often have access to an electronic form of the article as well as the usual citation information such as author, title, and abstract. The strategy for searching these specific Web sites is similar to a Google search, but the information returned is only from that association Web site. The advantage is that the search is highly focused, but the disadvantage is that you only retrieve information prepared by that professional association. However, a search of a specific association Web site yields documents that you might not be able to retrieve with other search engines, such as information on professional ethics, clinical practice guidelines, and position statements (AAA, n.d.; ASHA, n.d.).

Highwire Press is a search engine and Web host for on-line journals produced as a service of Stanford University Libraries (Stanford University, n.d.). Highwire Press produces Web sites for over 1000 journals in the biological, medical, physical, and social sciences. According to information on the Highwire Web site, over 1,800,000 full text versions of articles are available without a subscription. A search of the term *audiology* via Highwire Press yielded more than 4500 articles in audiology and speech-language pathology journals (e.g., *American Journal of Audiology, American Journal of Speech-Language Pathology*), as well as in journals in medical science (e.g., *Archives of Otolaryngology, Journal of the American Medical Association*, and *Pediatrics*). A search of the term *speech pathology* yielded more than 18,800 articles.

Google Scholar is a final search tool that you can access via the Web without a subscription (About Google Scholar, 2007). Google Scholar is a specialized search service provided by Google that is designed to search the professional literature from many disciplines. Although a search constructed for Google Scholar looks very similar to one for the general version of Google, the content searched is very different. A general Google search returns a wide variety of content including information from Web sites with primarily a commercial purpose. On the other hand, Google Scholar searches within a narrower body of information with an emphasis on articles in peer-reviewed journals, books from academic publishers, and content from the Web sites of professional associations and universities (About Google Scholar, 2007). Google Scholar provides some valuable tools that might help you refine or extend your search. To find the most recent publications on a topic, select either the option Recent Articles when displaying results or use the date option on the advanced search page. Researchers also have the option to restrict their searches to a particular journal or a particular subject area (Advanced Scholar Search Tips, 2007). One very helpful tool is the Cited By option. If a Google Scholar search uncovers a particularly appropriate article, you can quickly identify additional articles where the first article was cited and included in the reference list. Citation searching is an efficient way to find recent information on a specific topic and, therefore, is covered in more detail in a following section. Because Google Scholar is a free search service with several helpful features, an example search using this search engine is included in the Appendix.

One on-line search engine, the *Communication Sciences and Disorders Dome* or ComDisDome, is specialized for audiologists and speech-language pathologists (Content Scan, 2006). An advantage of using a tool such as the ComDisDome is that your searches should be more efficient, because the Dome only scans content in speech, language, and hearing sciences. Thus, you should retrieve fewer irrelevant articles, compared to other search engines such as Google Scholar, even when using the same search terms (Content Scan, 2006). One of the unique features of the Dome is that once you complete a topic search, you can sort the results to view just journal articles, dissertations, and Web sites. Researchers can search the ComDisDome database via CSA Illumina (ProQuest, 2008), a search service provided via site licenses to colleges, universities, and other institutions. Because the ComDisDome database is designed for audiologists and speech-language pathologists, we include an example Dome search in the Appendix.

ScienceDirect is a premium service usually licensed by institutions such as colleges and universities (ScienceDirect Info, 2007). ScienceDirect includes journals in life and health sciences, as well as physical and social sciences. A search with Science-Direct includes the Medline database and often PubMed and ScienceDirect yield similar search results. An advantage of ScienceDirect is that the site includes full text versions of journal articles. However, you will only be able to access the journals included in your institution's subscription.

We included the *OhioLink Library Catalog* because this on-line catalog provides a means to search within books to identify specific chapters on your topic (Ohio Library and Information Network, 2007). Sometimes books are collections of chapters by different authors. The individual chapters, although all on related topics, can have very different titles. Thus, to find information on a specific topic within books, you need to be able to search the table of contents. OhioLink is a search engine that lets you accomplish this. The database for OhioLink includes the holdings in college and university libraries in Ohio, as well as the State Library of Ohio. When you search OhioLink for book chapters, keep in mind that the search returns results with any of your search terms unless you specify otherwise. As a test I searched the terms [motor learning principles] and retrieved 107 book citations. Several of the books included chapters with my terms in three different chapters. Notably, the records were organized from the most to least relevant, and books with all three terms in their titles were listed first. However, to eliminate some of the irrelevant citations, I searched again but placed the terms *motor learning* in quotation marks ["motor learning" principles]. This search yielded only 34 of the most relevant records.

Often current research is available in a doctoral dissertation before publication in a peer reviewed journal. The on-line *ProQuest Dissertations and Theses Database* is one way to find a doctoral dissertation on your topic (UMI Dissertation Publishing, 2008). Most university libraries provide access to this database.

When you begin a literature search, one or more of these on-line search services is a good starting point. However, you might miss some references if you rely entirely on an electronic search. For example, a journal might not be included in the database you search or the terms you searched might not retrieve an important article. A simple supplemental strategy is to *browse the key journals* in your field. Many publishers make the tables of contents for their journals available on their Web sites, and sometimes researchers enjoy a trip to their library to spend time browsing the current issues of their favorite journals. For example, the PubMed database does not include articles from the *Journal of Medical Speech-Language Pathology*. Once, when preparing a presentation on evidence based practice, I searched for articles on treatment of childhood apraxia using Pub-Med, ERIC, and other search engines. Although the searches uncovered several articles, an article by Strand and Debertine (2000) on integral stimulation treatment never appeared. However, I knew about the article because of browsing issues of the *Journal of Medical Speech-Language Pathology* where this article was published.

Another good supplemental strategy is to *find a bibliography or review article* on your topic, or to check the references from a previous research report. The intent of a bibliography is to provide a list of all of the important work on a particular topic, and sometimes a bibliography includes annotations or brief descriptions of the articles as well. The authors of review articles also cover all of the important work on a topic but present an organized narrative and interpretation of the work. By checking the reference lists prepared by other authors, you can be more certain that you found all of the key work on your topic.

A final strategy for finding information on a topic is to complete a *citation search* for articles that cite a source you already found. Let's consider some graduate students who have an interest in the topic of word production theories. They read a review article on the topic, "Models of Word Production," by Levelt (1999), but the article was several years old and the students wanted to find more recent information. These students could conduct a citation search to identify authors who cited Levelt in their articles. Earlier we discussed the fact that Google Scholar provides a tool for conducting a citation search. The students decided to search the title of Levelt's review, "Models of Word Production," in Google Scholar.[1] This search revealed that more than 90 articles included Levelt in their reference list and allowed the students to find the most recent work on the topic of word production models.

The *Science Citation Index* and *Social Sciences Citation Index* were the classic tools for completing a citation search. Currently, you can access the contents of the *Science Citation Index* from 1900 to the present or the contents of the *Social Sciences Citation Index* from 1956 to the present by using the *Web of Science* on-line search tool (Thompson Corporation, 2006). You need a subscription to use the *Web of Science*, but many major university libraries have an institutional subscription. Although the unique uses of *Web of Science* involve searches for articles that cite other published work, you also can complete general searches such as those you would conduct on PubMed or ERIC (Thompson Corporation, 2006).

---

[1]If you want to search an exact phrase or title in Google or Google Scholar, place the phrase or title in quotations.

Designing a Search Strategy

Although researchers have many on-line tools to use when looking for previous research on their topics, the quality of the information they retrieve depends on how well they design their search strategy. Researchers want to be both thorough and efficient, so they want to retrieve all of the important information without a lot of irrelevant information. The starting point for most on-line literature searches is to decide on your *search terms*. Perhaps you are interested in treatment of speech production errors in children with hearing impairments. You might start designing a search strategy by identifying the key words in your topic—*treatment, speech production, children, hearing impairment*. If you only searched with one or two of the terms, you would retrieve too many articles, and much of what you retrieved would be irrelevant. Thus, researchers usually combine several terms when they conduct a literature search. In our example, if you only searched *treatment*, *children*, and *hearing*, you probably would retrieve many irrelevant sources. If you added the term *speech* to your search, you would narrow the topic and retrieve more relevant information. You also need to consider whether or not you need to add some terms to your search. Sometimes authors use different terms or synonyms to refer to a similar concept. For example, authors might use different terms for treatment, such as *intervention* or *therapy*. Sometimes a researcher is primarily interested in retrieving a certain type of article. This might be the case if you were searching for evidence-based practice information. If looking for a specific type of article, include that term in your search, such as *clinical trial, meta-analysis*, or *systematic review*. The different search engines provide tools for combining terms to nar-

row your search as well as ways to include synonyms. In this section, we discuss some general strategies for designing a search, and in the Appendix we show how these strategies are implemented in several search engines.

Many search tools use the logical operators AND, OR, and NOT from Boolean logic (APA, 2007; Silverman, 1998). Using the AND operator is a way to narrow your search. For example, *language intervention* and *hearing aids* are very broad topics that would yield an overwhelming number of sources. However, if you combine these terms with additional terms to narrow your search, such as *language intervention AND preschool AND children*, or *hearing aids AND preschool AND children*, you reduce the number of sources to a more manageable number. In some on-line search engines such as Google and Google Scholar, the plus sign (+) serves the same purpose as the AND from Boolean logic.

Using the OR operator broadens your search to retrieve sources that use a synonym for one of your terms. As noted previously, the term intervention has potential synonyms such as treatment or therapy. Thus, we might want to revise our example search for language intervention approaches as follows: *language AND (intervention OR treatment OR therapy) AND preschool AND children*. The NOT operator is useful when you retrieve many sources that are irrelevant for the same reason. For example, a researcher might be looking for information about treatment for fluent aphasia (*treatment AND fluent AND aphasia*) but finds many articles that focus on treatment for nonfluent aphasia. By using the NOT operator, the researcher could eliminate these irrelevant articles (*treatment AND fluent AND aphasia NOT non*).

Knowing how to use logical operators is helpful for any literature search, but many search engines have advanced search options that help you with this task. For example, Highwire Press has an additional search options feature that lets you enter terms and then select *any*, *all*, or *phrase* options. The any selection works like the OR operator, whereas the all selection works like the AND operator. The advanced search option for Google Scholar includes the descriptors *with all of the words*, *with at least one of the words*, and *without the words* that work like the logical operators AND, OR, and NOT. For some other on-line search tools, the advanced search option includes drop-down boxes for selecting the logical operators. You need to be careful when using the OR selection this way. Traditionally, terms that were synonyms were placed inside parentheses and then connected with OR [e.g., *speech AND (treatment OR intervention)*]. However, when making selections with the drop-down boxes, sometimes you inadvertently create a search that is very broad (such as *speech AND treatment OR intervention*). This latter search appears to retrieve all articles that have both the terms speech and treatment, as well as any article that has the term intervention.

Problems with grammatical variations on terms, such as *child, children, children's*, or *stutter, stutterer, stuttering*, can cause problems for some search engines. The PubMed search engine handles grammatical variations with its term matching capability. Using the OR operator is another way to handle grammatical variations (e.g., *child OR children OR children's*). However, some search engines allow you to use the *truncation operator* (*) to handle grammatical variations. If a search engine recognizes this operator, typing *child** or *stutter** would retrieve that term and any similar terms with additional letters (children, children's; stutterer, stuttering). You might check the on-line help option to determine

if the search tool you are using recognizes the truncation operator or implements this strategy in a different way.

Finally, many on-line search tools let you *set limits* on your search to reduce the number of sources you retrieve. Most search engines let you set a publication date when you conduct a search. Setting a minimum date of publication, such as only articles published from 2000 to the present, lets you conduct a slightly broader search while still retrieving a reasonable number of sources. Some other limits are specifying the language (articles written in English), the type of article (clinical trial, review), and the age of participants (adults, school-age children, preschool children).

The options available for the various on-line search engines are too numerous to cover thoroughly in this chapter. However, the Web sites for search engines such as Google Scholar, PubMed, ERIC, and ComDisDome all provide a help option. The help option gives explanations of how to construct a search in that particular search engine and how to use advanced search options to achieve better results.

Organizing and Documenting Your Literature Search

Once you have completed a search, how you use the evidence depends on whether you were conducting a search to find evidence to guide clinical practice, an interesting question to study, or background information and previous research on a research topic. If conducting a search for general clinical evidence, you might identify one or more meta-analyses or systematic reviews and read them to understand how the information relates to your clinical practice. Perhaps you need to include a summary of this evidence in your clinical documentation. If conducting a search for evidence on behalf of an individual client, you might select two or three articles that offer the highest quality evidence and most closely match your client's situation (Gallagher, 2002). After reading and evaluating this information, you might discuss your findings with the client or with family members.

If you conducted a literature search because you plan to write a research paper, you need to begin reading the articles, taking notes on content, and eventually writing content summaries to include in the introductory or review of literature section of your paper. Often an introduction and review of literature has a brief introduction and then a somewhat lengthier review of previous research. How much you write about the articles retrieved with the literature search depends on the type of paper. For example, a thesis or dissertation might be quite lengthy, and the introduction might be a few pages and the review literature 20 pages or more. The research reports in professional journals are more concise, and the introduction might be just a couple of paragraphs followed by several pages of literature review.

One way to organize the sources retrieved during a search is to develop a topic outline. This could include general topics such as background information, theoretical issues, methods of investigation, and previous research related to the topic. Usually authors discuss the previous research that is closest to their research question in the section before their statement of purpose or research questions. Sometimes the introduction and review of previous research includes information from more than one body of work. For example, researchers might be investigating a topic such as preschool children's attention and joint activity with peers when using a computer. How-

ever, the researchers planned to study this question with young children with communication disorders. Perhaps they could not find any previous research that covered all of these topics; however, they might find previous research that addressed some of these topics, such as children's attention in individual compared to joint activity, children's attention when using computers compared to other activities, or the use of computers in treatment of children with communication disorders. The topic outline for this review of literature might include subheadings for each of these categories of previous research. However you organize your review of literature, the general goals are to describe the broad problem, to establish the importance of the study, and to provide a topic-by-topic description of the relevant literature. Usually authors critique the existing research studies, noting any missing information or conflicting results. A good way to learn about organizing and summarizing information in a review of literature is to read the introductory section of several research reports. However, instead of just reading for comprehension, also pay attention to the topic organization and how the authors write about the studies they included in their review.

As discussed in the chapter on research ethics, authors need to carefully document their sources when they use the ideas or writing of another person. Usually this documentation includes citing the source in the text of a paper as well as listing the source in a reference list. A style manual, such as the *Publication Manual of the American Psychological Association*, 5th edition provides guidelines for citing sources in an appropriate way and preparing a reference list (APA, 2001; 2005). Many journals in communication sciences and disorders follow APA style, so we will review some of the most common citation and reference styles.

Authors should include a citation whenever they use a direct quote from another source or when they paraphrase another author's ideas. In APA style, the text citation includes the author(s) and year, and if a direct quote, it also includes the page number. A quotation is placed in quotation marks if it is less than 40 words and in an indented text block if 40 words or more (APA, 2001). A good writer uses direct quotes from other authors sparingly, so in the examples below we focus on paraphrases and short quotations.

Example 1: Paraphrase from a single source

Fu and Galvin (2006) used simulated speech to investigate cochlear implant users' ability to understand speech over the telephone.

Example 2: Paraphrase from a single source

Speaking rate at an early age is one possible predictor of a future reading disability in children with a positive family history (Smith, Roberts, Smith, Locke, & Bennett, 2006).

In the first example the source is cited within the text of the sentence, whereas in the second example the source is cited within parentheses at the end of the sentence (APA, 2001). Future citations of the study by Fu and Galvin always would include both authors. However, future citations of the Smith, Roberts, Smith, Lock, and Bennett study would be in the form Smith et al. (2006) because this report had three or more authors (APA, 2001). The APA style for including a short quote from another source is similar to the paraphrase, except that you need to place the information inside quotation marks and include the page number for the quote.

Example 3: Short quote from another source

With regard to children with closed head injury, Hay and Moran (2005, p. 333) noted " . . . it is important to be able to evaluate how they will cope with the communicative, social, and academic demands that will be placed on them with a return to their normal environment."

Example 4: Short quote from another source

With regard to children with closed head injury, " . . . it is important to be able to evaluate how they will cope with the communicative, social, and academic demands that will be placed on them with a return to their normal environment" (Hay & Moran, 2005, p. 333).

Finally, researchers also need to prepare a reference list for their papers. Although you could wait until finishing your paper to complete this list, you might find it helpful to generate the reference list in an ongoing way and to add an entry each time you cite a source. The APA style manual includes specific guidelines for what information to include and how to format your reference list. A reference list entry generally includes the author(s), date of publication, and title. If the source is a book, the entry also includes publisher information. If the source is a journal article, the entry includes the journal title, as well as volume and page numbers. For information retrieved from a Web site, the entry includes the date you viewed the information as well as the Web site address. Examples of entries for journal articles, a book, a chapter in edited books, and a Web site illustrate the different formats for these common types of sources.

Example 5: Entry for a journal article

McFadden, T. U. (1998). Sounds and stories: Teaching phonemic awareness in interactions around text. *American Journal of Speech-Language Pathology*, 7(2), 5-13.

Example 6: Entry for a journal article from an on-line source

Smith, D. (2003). Five principles for research ethics [Electronic version]. *Monitor on Psychology, 34*(1), 56.

Example 7: Entry for a book

Goldsworthy, C. L. (1998). *Sourcebook of phonological awareness activities: Children's classic literature.* San Diego, CA: Singular.

Example 8: Entry for a chapter in an edited book

Blachman, B. A. (1989). Phonological awareness and word recognition: Assessment and intervention. In A. G. Kamhi & H. Catts (Eds.), *Reading disabilities: A developmental perspective* (pp. 133–158). Boston: Allyn and Bacon.

Example 9: Entry for a Web site document

Centers for Disease Control and Prevention. (1997). *CDC procedures for protection of human research participants.* Retrieved October 11, 2007, from http://www.cdc.gov/od/foia/manuals/procphrp.pdf

Summary

In this chapter we focused on the skills needed to complete a literature search, cite information, and complete a reference list. The term *information literacy* is often used to refer to the skills researchers need to complete a literature search. Audiologists and speech-language pathologists have many reasons to search professional literature both in their clinical and research roles. Clinically, they might need to find answers to clinical or evidence-based practice questions. As a researcher, they might want to find interesting problems to study, previous research on a topic, background information on a topic, relevant information from other studies, or procedures and outcomes measures. One of the most efficient ways to conduct a literature search is to use an on-line search engine. Audiologists and speech-language pathologists can choose from among many Web-based search tools, such as ERIC, PubMed, Google Scholar, and ComDisDome.

Another aspect of information literacy is knowing how to design an appropriate search strategy. Audiologists and speech-languages pathologists need to know how to identify the key terms for their search, how to determine possible synonyms for these terms, and how to combine these terms to complete a thorough and efficient literature search. The various on-line search engines provide search aids to help you combine terms, set date limits, and retrieve specific types of articles.

Finally, researchers need to know the appropriate way to cite or attribute ideas to their appropriate sources and how to generate a reference list. Usually, a publication such as a journal or book uses a particular style for citing sources and formatting a reference list. Journals in the field of communication sciences and disorders commonly use the style described in the *Publication Manual of the American Psychological Association*, 5th edition (APA, 2001).

Review Questions

1. What term refers to the skills associated with finding, evaluating, summarizing, and using information?

2. List three reasons why audiologists and speech-language pathologists conduct searches of professional literature.

3. What is the most efficient way to search the professional literature?

4. If your study focused on children and/or educational topics, what search engine is the best choice for your search?

5. List three search engines that you can use for free.

6. If your research topic focused on adults and/or medical issues, what search engine is the best choice for your search?

7. What free search engine provides a way to complete a citation search?

8. What is the role of the AND operator in Boolean logic?

9. Identify the combination of terms that would retrieve fewer sources or would be narrower.
   a. *speech OR language OR hearing*
   b. *speech AND language AND hearing*

10. Identify the combination of terms that would retrieve more sources or would be broader.
    a. *delay OR disorder OR impairment*
    b. *delay AND disorder AND impairment*

11. Which of the following statements is true?

   a. In APA style you cite the source of an idea in a paraphrase by using a footnote at the end of your paper.
   b. In APA style you cite the source of an idea by including the author and year in your paragraph.

12. What information do you usually include when listing a journal article in your reference list?

Learning Activities

1. Think of a topic for a literature search. Choose two or more of the following databases and conduct a search on that topic. Modify your search by adding an additional term to narrow your search and by choosing one or more synonyms for your search terms to broaden your search.
   a. Education Resources Information Center (ERIC)
   b. PubMed
   c. American Speech-Language-Hearing Association Web site
   d. American Academy of Audiology Web site
   e. Highwire Press
   f. Google Scholar
   g. ComDisDome

2. Visit one of the on-line writing centers such as one of the two listed below. Read the information about paraphrasing and citing information from another author's work.
   a. UW-Madison Writing Center at http://www.wisc.edu/writing/Handbook/index.html

b. Purdue OWL at http://owl.english.purdue.edu/owl/resource/563/01/

3. Each of the following entries in a reference list has an error in format. Identify the error. A style reference such as the *Publication Manual of the American Psychological Association*, 5th edition (APA, 2001) or *Concise Rules of APA Style* (APA, 2005) would be helpful for this task.

Clements, D. H., & Nastasi, B. K. (1993). Electronic media and early childhood education. In B. Spodek (Ed.), *Handbook of research on the education of young children.* New York, NY: Macmillan (pp. 251–274).

Cook, A. M., & Hussey, S. M. (1995). *Assistive Technologies: Principles and Practice.* St. Louis, MO: Mosby.

Fey, M. E., & Cleave, P. L. (1990). Early language intervention. *Seminars in Speech and Language,* 165–181.

Haugland, S. W. (1995). Classroom Activities Provide Important Support to Children's Computer Experiences. *Early Childhood Education Journal, 23,* 99–100.

Haugland, S. W., & Wright, J. L. (1997). *Young children and technology: A world of discovery.* Allyn and Bacon: Boston.

Liu, M. (1996). An exploratory study of how pre-kindergarten children use the interactive multimedia technology: Implications for multimedia software design. *Journal of Computing in Childhood Education,* 7.

Rowland & Scott (1992). Promoting language and literacy for young children through computers. *Journal of Computing in Childhood Education, 3,* 55–61.

Shriberg et al. (1989). Tabletop versus microcomputer-assisted speech management: Stabilization phase. *Journal of Speech and Hearing Disorders, 54,* 233–248.

References

About Google Scholar. (2007). Retrieved January 7, 2008, from http://scholar.google.com intl/en/scholar/about.html

Advanced Scholar search tips. (2007). Retrieved January 7, 2008, from http://scholar.google.com/intl/en/scholar/refinesearch.html

American Academy of Audiology. (n.d.). *Publications & strategic documents.* Retrieved January 7, 2008, from http://www.audiology.org/publications/

American Library Association. (2006, July). *Introduction to information literacy.* Retrieved January 5, 2008, from http://www.ala.org/ala/acrl/acrlissues/acrlinfolit/infolitoverview/introtoinfolit/introinfolit.cfm

American Psychological Association. (2001). *Publication manual of the American Psychological Association* (5th ed.). Washington, DC: Author.

American Psychological Association. (2005). *Concise rules of APA style.* Washington, DC: Author.

American Psychological Association. (2007). *Search tips: A primer on Boolean logic.* Retrieved January 8, 2008, from http://www.apa.org/psycinfo/training/boolean.html

American Speech-Language-Hearing Association. (2004). *Preferred practice patterns for the profession of speech-language pathology.* Retrieved December 1, 2007, from http://www.asha.org/docs/html/PP2004-00191.html#sec1.2

American Speech-Language-Hearing Association. (2006). *Preferred practice patterns for the profession of audiology.* Retrieved December 1, 2007, from http://www.asha.org/docs/html/PP2004-00191.html#sec1.2

American Speech-Language-Hearing Association. (n.d.). *ASHA publications.* Retrieved January 7, 2008, from http://www.asha.org/about/publications/

Ask. (2008). *Help central.* Retrieved January 5, 2008, from http://about.ask.com/en/docs/about/help_central.shtml

Content Scan. (2006). *The web is for everyone, the Dome is for you.* Retrieved January 7, 2008, from http://www.comdisdome.com/thedome.jsp?_payprogids=defaultProgram&_JSESSIONID=78518087FC7619600D712BCB53EDF896

CSA Illumina. (n.d.). *About CSA.* Retrieved January 8, 2008, from http://www.csa.com/

Fu, Q.-J., & Galvin, J. J., III. (1996). Recognition of simulated telephone speech by cochlear implant users. *American Journal of Audiology, 15,* 127–132.

Gallagher, T. M. (2002). Evidence-based practice: Applications to speech-language pathology. *Perspectives on Language Learning and Education, 9*(1), 2–5.

Google. (2007). *Google help center.* Retrieved January 3, 2008, from http://www.google.com/help/basics.html

Gordon-Salant, S., Fitzgibbons, P. J., & Friedman, S. A. (2007). Recognition of time-compressed and natural speech with selective temporal enhancements by young and elderly listeners. *Journal of Speech, Language, and Hearing Research, 50,* 1181–1193.

Hay, E., & Moran, C. (2005). Discourse formulation in children with closed head injury. *American Journal of Speech-Language Pathology, 14,* 324–336.

Institute of Education Sciences. (n.d.). *Education Resources Information Center.* Retrieved December 1, 2007, from http://www.eric.ed.gov/

Levelt, W. J. M. (1999). Models of word production. *Trends in Cognitive Sciences, 3*(6), 223–232.

Ma, E. E.-M., & Yiu, E. M.-L. (2001). Voice activity and participation profile: Assessing the impact of voice disorders on daily activities. *Journal of Speech, Language, and Hearing Research, 44,* 511–524.

Marton, K., & Schwartz, R. G. (2003). Working memory capacity and language processes in children with specific language impairment. *Journal of Speech, Language, and Hearing Research, 46,* 1138–1153.

National Center for Biotechnology Information. (2007, September 19). *PubMed overview.* Retrieved January 7, 2008, from http://www.ncbi.nlm.nih.gov/entrez/query/static/overview.html

National Center for Biotechnology Information. (2007, December 19). *PubMed help.* Retrieved January 7, 2008, from http://www.ncbi.nlm.nih.gov/books/bv.fcgi?rid=helppubmed.chapter.pubmedhelp

Ohio Library and Information Network. (2007). Retrieved January 7, 2007, from http://www.ohiolink.edu/

Patten, M. L. (2007). *Understanding research methods: An overview of the essentials* (6th ed.). Glendale, CA: Pyrczak.

ProQuest. (2008). *CSA Illumina: Databases & collections.* Retrieved January 8, 2008, from http://www.csa.com/e_products/databases-collections.php

Schardt, C., & Mayer, J. (2004). *Introduction to evidence-based medicine.* Retrieved January 8, 2007, from http://www.hsl.unc.edu/services/tutorials/ebm/index.htm. Duke University Medical Center Library and Health Sciences Library, UNC-Chapel Hill.

ScienceDirect info. (2007). Retrieved January 7, 2008, from http://www.info.sciencedirect.com/

Silverman, F. H. (1998). *Research design and evaluation in speech-language pathology and audiology: Asking and answering questions* (4th ed.). Englewood Cliffs, NJ: Prentice Hall.

Smith, A. B., Roberts, J., Smith, S. L., Locke, J. L., & Bennett, J. (1996). Reduced speaking rate as an early predictor of reading disability. *American Journal of Speech-Language Pathology, 15,* 289–297.

Stanford University. (n.d.). *Highwire Press: A brief introduction.* Retrieved January 7, 2008, from http://highwire.stanford.edu/about/intro.dtl

Strand, E. A., & Debertine, P. (2000). The efficacy of integral stimulation treatment with developmental apraxia of speech. *Journal of Medical Speech-Language Pathology, 8*(4), 295–300.

Thompson Corporation. (2006). *Web of Science: Tutorial* (v7.8). Retrieved January 7, 2008, from http://scientific.thomson.com/tutorials/wos7/wos7tut1.html

UMI Dissertation Publishing. (2008). Retrieved January 7, 2007, from http://il.proquest.com/products_umi/dissertations/

World Health Organization. (2001). *International classification of functioning, disability and health.* Geneva, Switzerland: Author.

APPENDIX

Electronic Literature Search

The activities in this section provide some practice with Web-based search engines for those who have limited experience conducting on-line searches. For this demonstration, we will conduct an evidence-based practice search for the sample questions from Chapter 3. These questions are listed below:

1. Will minimal pair phonological treatment, provided for two 30-minute individual treatment sessions per week for 16 weeks, produce a 20% gain in percentage of consonants correct in spontaneous speech for a 5-year-old child with a moderately severe speech production disorder?
2. Will early detection of hearing loss and amplification fitting prior to 6 months of age result in age-appropriate scores on a test of expressive and receptive language at age 2 for a child with a severe hearing loss, when provided without additional speech and language intervention?

We will conduct the same search using four different search tools, ERIC, PubMed, Google Scholar, and ComDisDome. Our goal will be to retrieve somewhere between 25 and 75 sources. This is a somewhat arbitrary number and we certainly would be comfortable with a few more or less. However, if you retrieve too few, your search might be too narrow or you missed some synonyms. If you retrieve too many, you could go through a large number of sources to find what you want, but that is inefficient. If you have a computer with a relatively current Web browser and an Internet connection, you should be able to access ERIC, PubMed, and Google Scholar without any problems. These three search engines are free services. ComDisDome is a commercial product provided for a fee. You might check your institution's library or information services department to determine if you have a site license for this product.

Part 1: Identify Key Terms and Possible Synonyms

1. The first step is to identify key terms from your evidence-based practice or research question. These terms form the basis for your search.
   a. Key terms for question 1 might include *minimal pair, phonological, treatment, 5-year-old* or *child, speech production disorder*.
   a. Key terms for question 2 might include *early detection, hearing loss, amplification, expressive language, receptive language, child*.

2. The next step is to decide which of the key terms to include in your initial search strategy.
   a. For question 1, you might use *phonological, treatment, child*, and *disorder*. Using a specific treatment approach like *minimal pair* might narrow the search too much, as would including a specific age group. The term *speech production* overlaps with *phonological*, so you could just use the term *disorder*.

b. For question 2, you might use *early detection, hearing loss, language*. The term *child* overlaps with *early detection*, and *amplification* overlaps with *hearing loss*. You could consider adding the term *longitudinal* because you are looking for follow-up studies.

3. The third step is to identify possible synonyms for the terms you picked.
   a. For question 1, several terms might have synonyms or grammatical variations. Possible synonyms include: (a) *treatment, intervention, therapy*; (b) *disorder, delay, impairment*. Terms with possible grammatical variations include *child* and *phonological*. You will need to decide after trying the search whether or not to consider articulation treatment and/or articulation disorders.
   b. For question 2, some terms might have synonyms such as: (a) *early detection, early identification, early intervention*, (b) *hearing loss, hearing impairment*, and (c) *longitudinal, follow up*. You will need to decide after trying a search if you want to include *speech* as an alternative for *language*.

Part 2: Complete an ERIC Search

Decide whether to search on question 1 or question 2. The steps for both questions are the same.

Question 1

1. Begin by going to the ERIC Web site at http://www.eric.ed.gov/

2. Look for the Advanced Search option toward the top of the page and click on it.

3. In the Advanced Search you should see the words *Search for* followed by three fields where you can enter terms.

4. Begin with a basic search by typing *phonological* in the first box, *treatment* in the second box, *child* in the third box. We need another row so click on Add Another Row and type *disorder* in the box that appears.

5. Click on the Search button to start your search.

6. This search returned only a few results, but we already planned to revise it by using synonyms and grammatical variations.

7. In the window with your search results, click on Back to Search, so you can revise the search.

8. ERIC supports truncation so we will truncate the term *phonological* by replacing it with *phono** and truncate *child* by typing *child**. You might want to click on the Search button again just to see how truncating affected the number of results you retrieved.

9. If you decided to try the previous modification, click on Back to Search. Further revise your search by adding synonyms. In the box with *treatment*, type *treatment OR intervention OR therapy*. In the box with *disorder*, type *disorder* OR delay* OR impairment**.

10. Click on the Search button again. This time you should retrieve many more results. Probably you retrieved too many articles with this search strategy.

11. Because we retrieved too many articles, let's limit the search by searching only for relatively recent publications. Click on Back to Search and look for the option Publication Date. Reset the From date to a more recent date, such as

1995. This time you should retrieve fewer results.

12. Scroll down the list to view the articles you retrieved. To see the full abstract of an article, click on Show Full Abstract. You might experiment with other options in ERIC or develop a search strategy for another topic. Then, try this same search in a different Web-based search tool.

Question 2

1. Begin by going to the ERIC Web site at http://www.eric.ed.gov/
2. Look for the Advanced Search option toward the top of the page and click on it.
3. In the Advanced Search you should see the words *Search for* followed by three fields where you can enter terms.
4. Begin with a basic search by typing *early* in the first box, *detection* in the second box, *hearing loss* in the third box. We need another row so click on Add Another Row and type *language* in the box that appears.
5. Click on the Search button to start your search.
6. This search returned only a few results, but we already planned to revise it by using synonyms and grammatical variations.
7. In the window with your search results, click on Back to Search, so you can revise your search.
8. ERIC supports truncation so we will truncate the term *detection*. It could have grammatical variations. Let's truncate the term *detection* as *detect** and one of its synonyms as *ident** (see below for the synonyms).
9. Revise your search by adding synonyms. In the box with *detection*, type

detect* OR ident* OR intervention. In the box with *hearing loss*, type *hearing AND (loss OR impairment)*. Be sure to place *loss OR impairment* in parentheses.

10. Click on the Search button again. This time you should retrieve many more results. Probably you retrieved too many articles with this search strategy.

11. Because we retrieved too many articles, let's limit the search by searching only for relatively recent publications. Click on Back to Search and look for the option Publication Date. Reset the From date to a more recent date, such as 2000. This time you should retrieve fewer results.

12. Scroll down the list to view the articles you retrieved. To see the full abstract of an article, click on Show Full Abstract. You might experiment with other options in ERIC or develop a search strategy for another topic. Then, try this same search in a different Web-based search tool.

Part 3: Complete a PubMed Search

You probably want to search the same question on ERIC and PubMed, so you can compare results. The steps for question 1 and 2 are the same.

Question 1

1. Begin by going to the PubMed Web site at http://www.ncbi.nlm.nih.gov/PubMed/
2. Look for the line Search PubMed For followed by a long box.

3. Click on the box and begin by typing *phonological AND treatment AND child AND disorder* in the box.
4. Click on the Go button to start your search.
5. The search returned quite a few results. To view the abstracts for the articles listed, click on the author row (it should be highlighted as a link).
6. PubMed has a term matching feature that handles the grammatical variations for some terms fairly well. It also supports truncation, although use of a truncation operator (*) turns off term matching. We will use truncation to make sure we retrieve all of the relevant literature. This time type *phonolog* AND treatment AND child* AND disorder** in the search box. Click on the Go button again just to see how this affected the number of results you retrieve.
7. You probably retrieved more sources by using truncation. Further revise your search by adding synonyms. This time type *phonology* AND (treatment OR intervention OR therapy) AND child* AND (disorder* OR delay OR impairment)* in the search box.
8. Click on the Go button again. Again you should retrieve more results. Probably you retrieved too many articles when you did this search.
9. Because we retrieved too many articles, let's limit the search by searching only for relatively recent publications. Click on the Limits tab toward the top of page and look for the option Published in the Last. Change this option to *5 years*. Let's set a Language limit also. Scroll down until you see the Languages box on the left side of the page. Place a check mark beside English. We also retrieved some articles that focused on reading and literacy. We can eliminate these by adding *NOT literacy NOT*

reading to our search—*phonolog* NOT literacy NOT reading AND (treatment OR intervention OR therapy) AND child* AND (disorder* OR delay OR impairment)*. This time when you click on Go you should retrieve fewer results.
10. You might experiment with other options for Limits in PubMed or develop a search strategy for another topic. Afterward, repeat this same search in either Google Scholar or ComDisDome.

Question 2

1. Begin by going to the PubMed Web site at http://www.ncbi.nlm.nih.gov/PubMed/
2. Look for the line Search PubMed For followed by a long box.
3. Click on the box and begin by typing *early AND detection AND hearing loss AND language* in the box.
4. Click on the Go button to start your search.
5. The search returned quite a few results. To view the abstracts for the articles listed, click on the author row (it should be highlighted as a link).
6. PubMed has a term matching feature that handles the grammatical variations for some terms fairly well. It also supports truncation, although use of a truncation operator (*) turns off term matching. We will use truncation to make sure we retrieve all of the relevant literature. This time type *early AND detect* AND hearing loss AND language*. Click on the Go button again just to see how this affected the number of results you retrieve.
7. You probably retrieved more sources by using truncation. Further revise your search by adding synonyms. This time type *early AND (detect* OR identif**

OR intervention) AND hearing AND (loss OR impairment) AND language in the search box.

8. Click on the Go button again. This time you should retrieve many more results. Probably you retrieved too many articles when you did this search.

9. Because we retrieved so many articles, let's limit the search by searching only for the most recent publications. Click on the *Limits* tab toward the top of page and look for the option Published in the Last. Change this option to *5 years*. Let's set a Language limit also. Scroll down until you see the Languages box on the left side of the page. Place a check mark beside English. We also retrieved some articles that focused on cochlear implants and otitis media. We can eliminate these by adding *NOT cochlear NOT otitis* to our search—*early AND (detect* OR identif* OR intervention) NOT cochlear NOT otitis AND hearing AND (loss OR impairment) AND language*. This time when you click on Go you should retrieve fewer results.

10. You might experiment with other options for Limits in PubMed or develop a search strategy for another topic. Afterward, repeat this same search in either Google Scholar or ComDisDome.

Part 4: Complete a Google Scholar Search

If you want to compare results, you should stay with the same question and terms you searched on ERIC and PubMed.

Question 1

1. Begin by going to the Google Scholar Web site at http://scholar.google.com/

2. Look for the Advanced Scholar Search option to the right of the search box and click on it.

3. In Advanced Scholar Search you should see the phrase *Find articles* followed by some phrases such as *with all the words*, *with the exact phrase*, and so forth. These are followed by text boxes where you can enter terms.

4. Begin with a basic search by typing *phonological treatment child disorder* in the box following the phrase *with all the words*.

5. Click on the *Search Scholar* button to start your search.

6. You probably retrieved a very large number of sources (over 10,000).

7. Generally, Google Scholar returns many sources and you primarily need to narrow your search rather than add synonyms or grammatical variants. At the top of the window, click on Advanced Scholar Search. This will return you to the page where you enter search terms.

8. First, let's try to limit the search to just the titles of articles. Look for the phrase *where my words occur*. To the right of this, you should see the phrase *anywhere in the article*. Click on the arrow to the right of this phrase and select in the title of the article. Click on the Search Scholar button again. You probably found that this option severely narrowed your search.

9. Let's try some different options for narrowing the search. First, click on Advanced Scholar Search to return to the page where you enter search terms. Go to where my words occur and reset this to anywhere in the article.

10. Now limit the search to the most recent articles by entering the year 2000 in the first box following Date return articles published between. Also, let's limit the search by topic. Place check marks

in Biology, Life Sciences, and Environmental Sciences and Social Sciences, Arts, and Humanities. Finally, I noticed a few of the articles retrieved were about children who stutter and also about children with reading problems. We can eliminate these by typing words such as *stutter stuttering reading* following the phrase *without the words*.

11. Let's try the search again by clicking the Search Scholar button. We did retrieve fewer results (over 350) this time, but that still would be too many. However, Google Scholar prioritizes the sources and the most relevant should appear first in your list, so you should not have to view all 350 entries.

12. Finally, let's try the Google Scholar Cited by feature. Perhaps look for an article published in 2000 and addressing our topic of treatment of a 5-year-old child with a moderate-to-severe phonological disorder. Click on the Cited by link to find articles that included this one in their citations and references. You might experiment by trying other options to narrow this search such as using additional terms, or perhaps design a new search on a topic of your choice. If you have access to ComDisDome, you should try this same search with that tool as well.

Question 2

1. Begin by going to the Google Scholar Web site at http://scholar.google.com/

2. Look for the Advanced Scholar Search option to the right of the search box and click on it.

3. In Advanced Scholar Search you should see the phrase *Find articles* followed by some phrases such as *with all the words*, *with the exact phrase*, and so

forth. These are followed by text boxes where you can enter terms.

4. Begin with a basic search by typing *early detection hearing loss language* in the box following the phrase *with all the words*.

5. Click on the Scholar Search button to start your search.

6. You probably retrieved a very large number of sources (over 20,000).

7. Generally, Google Scholar returns many sources and you primarily need to narrow your search rather than add synonyms or grammatical variants. At the top of the window, click on Advanced Scholar Search. This will return you to the page where you enter search terms.

8. First, let's try to limit the search to just the titles of articles. Look for the phrase *where my words occur*. To the right of this, you should see the phrase *anywhere in the article*. Click on the arrow to the right of this phrase and select in the title of the article. Click on the Search Scholar button again. You probably found that this option severely narrowed your search.

9. Let's try some different options for narrowing the search. First, click on Advanced Scholar Search to return to the page where you enter search terms. Go to where my words occur and reset this to anywhere in the article.

10. Now limit the search to the most recent articles by entering the year 2003 in the first box following Date return articles published between. Also, let's limit the search by topic. Place check marks in Biology, Life Sciences, and Environmental Sciences and Social Sciences, Arts, and Humanities. Finally, I noticed a few of the articles retrieved were about children with otitis media and others covered a genetic etiology. We can eliminate these by typing words

such as *otitis media genetic gene* following the phrase *without the words*.

11. Let's try the search again by clicking the Search Scholar button. We did retrieve fewer results (over 1600) this time, but that still would be too many. However, Google Scholar prioritizes the sources and the most relevant should appear first in your list, so you should not have to view all 1600 entries.

12. Finally, let's try the Google Scholar Cited by feature. Perhaps look for an article published in 2003 that seems to be highly relevant to our topic. Click on the Cited by link to find articles that included this one in their citations and references. You might experiment by trying other options to narrow this search such as using additional terms, or perhaps design a new search on a topic of your choice. If you have access to ComDisDome, you should try this same search with that tool as well.

Part 5: Complete a ComDisDome Search

Hopefully you have had some success searching with tools such as ERIC, PubMed, and Google Scholar. If you decide to search ComDisDome too, I suggest you continue with the same question, either question 1 or question 2, so you can compare results.

Question 1

1. This tutorial is based on accessing ComDisDome through CSA Illumina. You will only be able to complete this

search if you have either institutional or personal access to this search service. Some institutions provide access through their own Web site. Otherwise you might log in at http://www.csa.com/csaillumina/login.php

2. Find the Advanced Search option and click on it.

3. In the Advanced Search you should see a series of text fields where you can enter terms.

4. Begin with a basic search by typing *phonological AND child* in the first box, *treatment* in the second box, and *disorder* in the third box.[2] Make sure you select AND as your Boolean operator.

5. Click on the Search button to start your search.

6. The search returned quite few results. To view the abstracts for the articles listed, click on the title (it should be highlighted as a link).

7. In the window with your search results, click on Advanced Search again to revise your search.

8. Even though we found many articles, we still want to be thorough. Try truncation to retrieve variations such as *phonology* or *children*. This time type *phonolog* AND child**, then *treatment* and finally *disord**. You might want to click on the Search button again just to see how truncating affected the number of results you retrieved.

9. You probably retrieved more sources by using truncation. Further revise your search by adding synonyms. In the box with *treatment*, type *treatment OR intervention*. In the box with *disorder*, type *disorder* OR delay* OR impairment**.

---

[2]If you use CSA Illumina to search ComDisDome, you might see three boxes across for OR terms, and three boxes down for AND terms.

10. Click on the Search button again. This time you should retrieve many more results. Probably you retrieved too many articles when you did this search.

11. Because we retrieved so many articles, let's limit the search by searching only for the most recent publications. Go back to Advanced Search and reset the from date to a more recent one, such as to 2003. Also, plan to view only the results for journal articles. This time you should retrieve fewer results.

12. You might further explore ComDis-Dome by designing a search strategy for another topic.

Question 2

1. This tutorial is based on accessing ComDisDome through CSA Illumina. You will only be able to complete this search if you have either institutional or personal access to this search service. Some institutions provide access through their own Web site. Otherwise you might log in at http://www.csa.com/csaillumina/login.php

2. Find the Advanced Search option and click on it.

3. In the Advanced Search, you should see a series of text fields where you can enter terms.

4. Begin with a basic search by typing *early AND detection* in the first box, *hearing loss* in the third box, and *language* in the third box. Make sure you select AND as your Boolean operator. (See the footnote for question 1 if you are using CSA Illumina.)

5. Click on the Search button to start your search.

6. The search returned quite few results. To view the abstracts for the articles listed, click on the title (it should be highlighted as a link).

7. In the window with your search results, click on Advanced Search again to revise your search.

8. Even though we found many articles, we still want to be thorough. Try truncation to retrieve variations on the term *detection*. This time type *early AND detect** in the first box. You might want to click on the Search button again just to see how truncating affected the number of results you retrieved.

9. You probably retrieved more sources by using truncation. Further revise your search by adding synonyms. In the box with *early*, type *early AND (detect* OR ident* OR intervention)*. In the box with *hearing loss*, type *hearing AND (loss OR impairment)*. Be sure to place *loss OR impairment* in parentheses.

10. Click on the Search button again. This time you should retrieve many more results. Probably you retrieved too many articles when you did this search.

11. Because we retrieved so many articles, let's limit the search by searching only for the most recent publications. Go back to Advanced Search and reset the from date to a more recent one, such as to 2003. Also plan to view only the results for journal articles. This time you should retrieve fewer results.

12. You might further explore ComDis-Dome by designing a search strategy for another topic.

CHAPTER 5

Nonexperimental Research Design

Identifying an interesting problem to study and turning that problem into an answerable research question are early steps in a process of systematic inquiry. If a literature search revealed only a few previous studies on the topic and none that fully answered the question, the next step is to gather original evidence. Before beginning this process, researchers decide on the best approach and then develop a detailed plan for conducting their research. This plan or *research design* might include information about identifying participants, assigning participants to groups, manipulating or measuring variables, and analyzing the findings (Trochim & Donnelly, 2007). In the design you also might specify when you will make your observations and what the participants will do.

A research design is your plan for answering a research question or testing a research hypothesis. Researchers decide on the particular features of a design based on the nature of their study. Although research studies generally share at least one similarity—a question that needs an answer—the way a researcher obtains answers could vary broadly from making observations in an unobtrusive way to exposing participants to different experimental manipulations. Experimental studies are those in which

researchers identify one or more factors that they will manipulate or control during the experiment. Nonexperimental studies are those in which researchers investigate existing conditions or differences without manipulating them (Patten, 2007). In this chapter we focus on nonexperimental designs, including qualitative research designs.

Nonexperimental Research Designs

The designs for nonexperimental studies typically include plans to observe and describe behaviors, to determine relationships among measures of different skills, or to compare persons with different characteristics. Some examples of nonexperimental approaches include descriptive studies such as surveys, case studies, opinion polls, and prevalence studies; relationship studies involving correlation and prediction, comparisons of existing groups to identify differences by age, presence of a disorder, socioeconomic status, and so forth; and causal-comparative studies that examine the impact of possible causal factors over time (Patten, 2007). In the next sections, we will cover several common nonexperimental designs and discussion their use in the field of communication sciences and disorders.

Survey Research

You might have personal experience with *survey research*. Perhaps a researcher asked you to complete a paper and pencil or telephone survey on some topic, such as your opinion on a certain product or on election issues. Survey research generally involves obtaining participants' responses to a series of questions, either through a written questionnaire or an interview (Trochim & Donnelly, 2007). Researchers might consider using a survey when they want to collect data that reflect opinions or reports of individual experiences and when they want to collect information from a relatively large number of participants (Writing Center at Colorado State University, 2008). When designing a survey, a researcher needs to decide on several components, such as those listed below:

1. Survey participants
2. Content of questions
3. Types of questions
4. Sequence of questions
5. Survey procedure (e.g., written or interview)

The subject matter of a survey is the most important factor to consider when deciding who should complete the survey. For example, if the survey focuses on consumer satisfaction with speech, language, or hearing services, the survey participants should be the persons who received those services rather than the audiologists and speech-language pathologists who provided the services. Sometimes researchers have choices regarding the most appropriate participants. For example, if a survey focuses on children's actions and attitudes toward peers with communication disorders, the survey participants could be the children or perhaps their teachers. Additionally, the researchers might decide to compare responses from different groups of participants. They might survey different age groups, different professions (audiologists, speech-language pathologists, speech-language-hearing scientists), persons in different geographic locations, and so forth.

The content of survey questions relates closely to the validity of the survey or the extent to which it covers the material professionals in the field would expect. Further, survey researchers also need to consider if they are asking for information their respondents know, if the wording of the questions elicits appropriately specific information, and if the terminology in the questions is familiar to respondents (Trochim & Donnelly, 2007). A survey can include several types of questions including yes/no, categorical response, rating scale, semantic differential, cumulative response, and open-ended formats (Trochim & Donnelly, 2007). Table 5–1 includes examples of each type of question.

In addition to making decisions about the kinds of questions to use, survey researchers also need to make decisions about the sequence of questions, as well as how to administer the questions to participants. Trochim and Donnnelly (2007) suggested that surveys should start with straightforward questions and present probing or difficult questions toward the end. In deciding whether to use a written survey or interview, researchers should consider the advantages and disadvantages of each approach. Advantages of written surveys include the possibility of displaying graphic or pictorial content, greater privacy for respondents, relatively low cost, and ability to recruit par-

Table 5–1. Examples of six different types of survey questions

Type of Question	Example
Yes/no	1. Are you currently employed as an audiologist or speech-language pathologist? (Circle one.) Yes No
Categorical response	2. What is your current class standing? (Place an X beside one.) ____ Freshman ____ Sophomore ____ Junior ____ Senior ____ Graduate
Rating scale	3. Evidence based practice will improve the quality of patient care in audiology and speech-language. Strongly Agree Neutral Strongly Disagree 1 2 3 4 5
Cumulative response	4. In the past month, I provided speech, language, or hearing services to adults or children with: (Place an X beside all that apply.) ____ articulation/phonological disorders ____ auditory processing disorders ____ conductive hearing loss ____ fluency disorders ____ language disorders ____ sensorineural hearing loss ____ voice disorders ____ other (_____)
Open-ended	5. In your opinion, what are the three most important issues facing the field of communication sciences and disorders?

ticipants from a wider geographic area. Advantages of interviews include being able to explain the survey and answer participant questions, modify questions and ask follow-up questions, and include respondents who do not read or write (Trochim & Donnelly, 2007).

Although survey research is not the most common form of research in communication sciences and disorders, it does have an important role. For example, professional associations such as the American Speech-Language-Hearing Association and the American Academy of Audiology conduct surveys on behalf of their membership (American Academic of Audiology [AAA], 2006; American Speech-Language-Hearing Association [ASHA], 2006a; ASHA, 2006b; ASHA, 2007). Surveys have also been published in professional journals on a variety of topics (e.g., Allen, Pettit, & Sherblom, 1991; Hoffman et al., 2005; Roseberry-McKibbin, Brice, & O'Hanlon, 2005; Schwartz & Drager, 2008; Tharpe, Fino-Szumski, & Bess, 2001).

Case Studies

Often audiologists and speech-language pathologists encounter unique and interesting cases in their clinical practice. For example, a speech-language pathologist might complete a speech and language evaluation of a child with a rare genetic disorder. Perhaps, a search of the professional literature revealed little if any information about the communication abilities of persons with this disorder. An audiologist might complete hearing evaluations of workers and initiate a program to reduce industrial noise exposure at a manufacturing site. A search of the professional literature revealed very limited information on the unique challenges that emerged in this particular industrial setting. Both of these examples are situations that could lead to an interesting *case study*. Usually, when we think of case study research, we think of a descriptive study of an individual person. However, case studies also can be descriptive studies of other "units," such as an individual classroom, a particular acute care hospital, a specific industrial setting, and so forth. Also, researchers carrying out a case study could obtain either quantitative or qualitative data, and sometimes they choose both (Gillham, 2000; Hancock & Algozzine, 2006). For example, researchers might complete an in-depth evaluation using speech, language, and hearing tests that

yield numerical scores; and in addition, they could include interviews and direct observations. The data from the interviews and observations could be verbal in nature, such as direct quotes from those interviewed, or detailed field notes describing the person's behavior in different situations.

In designing a plan for a case study, researchers decide what measures, observations, and/or artifacts they want to collect. Two central features of most case studies are that the researchers use "multiple sources of evidence" (Gillham, 2000, p. 2) and that they study the case in typical, rather than experimental, settings (Gillham, 2000; Hancock & Algozzine, 2006). If the focus of a case study was a person with a communication disorder, you might gather information such as medical records and work samples (e.g., papers, drawings, or other documents); you might administer a series of speech, language, and hearing tests; you would probably interview the client and/or family as appropriate; you also would observe the person in some of his daily activities; and you almost always would obtain a spontaneous speech sample. If the focus of a case study was a unit such as a classroom or a medical facility, you could use many of the same methods, such as obtain records, review work samples, conduct interviews, or make observations. However, the nature of these data would be different. The records might include policy documents for the medical facility or the school district's curriculum document for that grade level. You probably would obtain work samples from many individuals, for instance collecting writing samples from several children.

If you searched the professional literature in the field of communication sciences and disorders and specifically looked for case studies, you would find many examples. In audiology and speech-language pathology, case studies often focus on descriptions of the characteristics and/or treatment of persons with various disorders, such as Asperger syndrome (Worth & Reynolds, 2008), autism and hyperlexia (Craig & Telfor, 2005), cerebral palsy and vision impairments (Blischak, 1995), cortical hearing impairment (Fowler, Kile, & Hecox, 2001), and progressive anomia (Ingles, Fisk, Passmore, & Darvesh, 2007).

Longitudinal Research

In *longitudinal research* an individual or group is followed for some amount of time. Researchers often combine longitudinal observation with other approaches such as longitudinal case studies, a correlation study with the intent of predicting future capabilities, or following different groups of children over time. Longitudinal research designs are common in studies of child development, including speech and language development. The amount of time covered in a longitudinal study varies considerably from relatively short studies of 1 to 2 years to very long-term studies of 25 or more years. Although longitudinal research often is nonexperimental, some experimental research does include long-term monitoring of treatment effects. Several of the case study examples identified above and some of the correlation/regression and group comparisons covered below are also longitudinal designs.

Correlation and Regression

Studies of relationships between two variables or among several variables and the kind of statistical analyses researchers perform are closely tied. If researchers are studying the relationship between two variables, then they usually perform a *correlation* analysis to determine strength of the relationship. If researchers are studying the relationship among several variables, they usually perform a *regression* analysis to determine the strength of the relationship and also which variables have the most predictive power. We will cover these statistical procedures in greater depth in Chapter 8. Our focus in this chapter is on the design of a study when the researcher's purpose is to investigate relationships.

Just like in designing other studies, researchers who are designing correlation and regression studies need to make decisions about who will participate, how to measure variables, and when to test the participants. In a correlation and regression study, a researcher recruits a group of participants and obtains two or more behavioral measures from each participant. This kind of study is nonexperimental because the researcher is measuring levels of performance that the participants have already achieved. The researcher is not training or manipulating the participants in any way to improve their performance. Usually when researchers conduct correlation studies, they have reason to believe that two variables share some kind of relationship. The researchers might believe that both variables reflect the same underlying trait, or they might even suspect that the two variables share a causal relationship. Unfortunately, correlation research *cannot* establish causality, only that two variables relate to one another in some unknown way.[1]

---

[1]Trochim and Donnelly (2007) cited an interesting example that illustrates why the presence of a correlation is *not* evidence of a causal relationship. According to these authors, researchers have discovered a correlation between the number of infants born in the United States and the number of roads built in Europe. Trochim and Donnelly pointed out that, although these two measures co-vary, there is no reason to assume a causal relationship. Rather, the two variables might both relate to a third unmeasured variable, such as the overall health of the world economy.

Another decision you need to make when planning correlation and regression research is whether you are interested in the immediate relationship between the variables or the long-term relationship. If researchers are interested in an immediate relationship, they need to complete all their observations or testing within a relatively short time. For example, if some speech-language pathologists had developed a shorter, more efficient way to test children's expressive and receptive language abilities, they would want to compare their new approach to one or more existing and well-accepted tests. However, they would need to administer both tests within a relatively short time; otherwise, the children's expressive and receptive language abilities could improve to the point where the two tests no longer tapped the same underlying skills.

Sometimes researchers want to know how variables relate over time and conduct a longitudinal correlation or regression study. Often the goal of this type of research is to discover measures that will predict future performance. In designing a *prediction study*, researchers need to decide how long they should follow their participants. Do they want to predict performance 1 year in the future or longer? Finally, researchers also need to decide how many measures they want to compare. They could design a study to investigate the relationship between just one predictor measure and one dependent measure (i.e., outcome measure). However, researchers often obtain several predictor measures and determine which variable or combination of variables produced the best results. Some interesting examples of correlation studies include several on the topic of predicting future language abilities or literacy skills (Foster-Cohen, Edgin, Champion, & Woodward, 2007; Hogan, Catts, & Little, 2005; Larney, 2002; Pankratz, Plante, Vance, & Insalaco, 2007; Reilly et al., 2007) and a recent study that focused on the relationship between the amount of noise exposure in an industrial setting and hearing loss (Rabinowitz, Galusha, Dixon-Ernst, Slade, & Cullen, 2007).

Group Comparisons

Group comparisons are another very common nonexperimental research approach in audiology and speech-language pathology. Although group comparisons can involve persons with normal communication, in communication sciences and disorders group comparisons usually involve persons with some type of communication disorder, such as a developmental language disorder, phonological disorder, aphasia, voice disorder, stuttering, sensorineural hearing loss, and so forth. When researchers design this type of study, they usually plan to test at least two different groups, such as persons with hearing loss and those with normal hearing, or children with phonological delays and those with normal phonological development. The researchers also identify some skill(s) they think will distinguish the two groups and decide on ways to measure those skills. Group comparisons have contributed to our understanding of the nature of speech, language, and hearing disorders, helped us better understand the impact of those disorders on development and participation, and provided clues into possible causes of communication disorders. Table 5–2 includes a list of some recent group comparison studies to illustrate the variety of topics addressed in the field of communication sciences and disorders.

Causal-Comparative Research

Identifying potential causal factors is an important avenue of study for audiologists and speech-language pathologists. Experi-

Table 5–2. A sample of recent group comparison studies in the field of communication sciences and disorders

Author(s)	Groups Compared	Measure(s)
Wetherell, Botting & Conti-Ramsden (2007)	Adolescents with specific language impairment (SLI) and typically developing peers	Narrative language
Goulandris, Snowling, & Walker (2000)	Adolescents with SLI and those with dyslexia	Reading and spelling
Estes, Evans, & Else-Quest (2007)	Children with SLI and typically developing peers	Nonword repetition
Archibald & Gathercole (2006)	Children with SLI and typically developing peers	Visuospatial memory
Bajaj, A. (2007)	Children who stutter and their typically developing peers	Oral narratives
Newman & Ratner (2007)	Adults who stutter and peers with fluent speech	Confrontation naming
Moeller et al. (2007)	Infants with hearing loss and infants with normal hearing	Vocalizations
Gordon-Salant, Fitzgibbons, & Friedman (2007)	Listeners who were elderly and those who were young	Speech recognition
Hicks, Bourland, & Tharpe (2002)	Children with hearing loss and peers with normal hearing	Listening effort
Horga & Liker (2006)	Persons who used cochlear implants, persons who were profoundly deaf with traditional hearing aids, and persons with normal hearing	Acoustic and perceptual measures of voice and speech

mental research designs are the strongest designs for establishing cause and effect relationships, but experimenting on research participants to determine the causes of communication disorders would be entirely unethical. For example, if researchers hypothesized that inadequate nutrition during infancy caused developmental problems later in childhood, they should not conduct an experiment in which they randomly assigned some infants to a group that received an adequate diet, and other infants to a group that received an inadequate diet.

Such an experiment would violate the basic principles of protection of human participants and expose the infants to substantial harm. When conducting experimental research is inappropriate, researchers have to identify an alternative approach for investigating the problem.

A *causal-comparative* study is one of the best alternatives for identifying potential causal factors. A causal-comparative study is similar to a group comparison study because the researchers investigate existing differences. However, one unique feature of causal-comparative studies is that researchers try to obtain several pieces of information about each participant. This feature is included in an attempt to identify possible "competing" causal factors in the participants' background and thus to strengthen the evidence for the causal variable under study. Often potential causal factors co-vary with other factors that also could cause speech, language, and hearing disorders. For example, poor medical care, inadequate housing, and poor nutrition are all factors associated with living in poverty. If researchers wanted to study poor nutrition as a causal factor in developmental disorders, they would have to consider if these other variables, poor medical care or inadequate housing, also could be causal factors. In a well-designed causal-comparative study, researchers obtain information about many variables, not just the variable under study, as a way to control for possible alternative explanations of their findings.

Researchers interested in conducting a causal-comparative study might decide to conduct either a retrospective study or a prospective study. In a retrospective causal-comparative study, researchers identify persons who vary on some condition (Patten, 2007). Usually this variable is the presence or absence of a medical or behavioral disorder, such as a speech, language, or hearing disorder. After identifying their participants, they obtain an extensive amount of information about their participants' medical history and family and social background (Patten, 2007). Usually this information will include the variable that is the focus of their study, as well as information about possible alternative causal explanations. For example, if the variable under study was poor nutrition, the researchers would also obtain information about other important factors such as medical complications at birth, number of siblings, parent income and/or

occupation, maternal and paternal education, and so forth.

Prospective causal-comparative studies share some similarities with retrospective studies. Researchers identify a potential causal factor, identify groups of persons who vary on this factor, and then obtain an extensive amount of information about their participants. However, the difference is that researchers in a prospective study identify their participants at the onset of the potential causal factor, and then follow them in a longitudinal research study. For example, if the causal factor was employment in an occupation where workers were exposed to environmental toxins, the researchers would identify the workers when they started their employment. They also would recruit a similar group who worked in an environment that was free of toxins. Over the course of their study, the researchers would periodically evaluate their participants to determine if any had developed a medical disorder, or perhaps communication disorder, and to determine if the occurrence of disorders was greater in the group exposed to the environmental toxins.

The reasoning behind a causal-comparative study is if a variable stands out as a potential cause after you control for many other variables, you have a strong argument for that variable as a cause of the disorder. Examples of causal-comparative research in communication sciences and disorders include studies of the developmental outcomes of low birth weight infants (Aram, Hack, Hawkins, Weissman, & Borawski-Clark, 1991; Foster-Cohen et al., 2007; Kilbride, Thorstad & Daily, 2004) and studies of the implications of recurrent otitis media for speech and language development (Roberts, Rosenfeld, & Zeisel, 2004; Shriberg, Friel-Patti, Flipsen, & Brown, 2000; Shriberg, Flipsen, et al., 2000). Although evidence from nonexperimental research is not sufficient to establish cause and effect relationships, the evidence is stronger if the researchers control for other variables. Thus, in the research focusing on low birth weight and otitis media, the researchers needed to obtain information about other potential causal factors such as medical complications at birth, quality of prenatal care, number of siblings, parent income and/or occupation, and maternal and paternal education, among others.

Qualitative Research

Qualitative research is a term that encompasses a number of research approaches that share several characteristics. The most obvious characteristic is how researchers record and report their findings. In qualitative research, the data typically include verbal statements such as direct quotes from participants, excerpts from writing samples, or detailed descriptions of behaviors (Gillham, 2000; Patten, 2007; Trochim & Donnelly, 2007). In contrast, the data in quantitative research are numeric in nature.

Another characteristic is that qualitative researchers usually rely on *inductive reasoning* to formulate a theory (Patten, 2007; Trochim & Donnelly, 2007). A qualitative researcher begins by gathering data in the form of oral or written statements, detailed descriptions, and so forth. After examining these specific forms of information, a qualitative researcher might identify trends or themes that emerged in the data and from these themes begin formulating a theory that fits the situation. That is, a qualitative researcher reasons from specific observations, to general trends, to an overarching theory. In contrast, quantitative researchers usually employ *deductive reasoning*, and begin with one or more theories about possible outcomes. They develop a specific hypothesis or prediction that stems from theory. Quantitative researchers design a study that yields specific information that either supports or refutes their predictions. Thus, they reason from the general theory, to a hypothesis or prediction, to gathering specific data to test their predictions.

Another important characteristic of qualitative research is that researchers study their participants in natural environments and situations. Qualitative researchers emphasize the need to understand the meaning of their participants' statements and behaviors and thus consider it vital to study participants in a natural, not artificial, context. In contrast, quantitative researchers usually set up an experimental or laboratory situation for their participants and ask their participants to perform activities they might not do in a typical day. Quantitative researchers emphasize the need to control the experimental situation so that all participants have very similar experiences during the study.

The emphasis on obtaining information from participants in their natural environments leads to another shared characteristic of qualitative studies. Qualitative researchers usually recruit only a small number of participants and then spend considerable time observing and interviewing these participants and reviewing artifacts such as writing and conversation samples (Patten, 2007). In contrast, quantitative researchers often recruit large numbers of participants, test them for a relatively short time in a laboratory setting, and then spend time organizing and analyzing data from fairly large groups.

Qualitative researchers also tend to be responsive to their participants, be open-ended in their research approach, and adjust their procedures as a situation dictates (Patten, 2007). Thus, a qualitative researcher would use a set of questions as an interview guide but would follow the participants' lead with regard to the topic of the interview. Similarly, they might plan to observe participants in certain situations but would be comfortable with a change in schedule and making observations in a different situation. In quantitative, experimental studies, the researchers' goal is to summarize findings across participants. Therefore, they need to obtain responses to the same questions from all participants and observe and test their participants in the same situations. Quantitative researchers have less freedom to modify their procedures to accommodate the unique needs of participants.

Although considering how qualitative research compares to quantitative research is helpful, in reality research often is neither purely qualitative nor purely quantitative (Damico & Simmons-Mackie, 2003; Gillham, 2000). In a study that is primarily qualitative, a researcher might count the number of statements that fit a certain theme, and in a study that is primarily quantitative, a researcher might take detailed field notes regarding participants' behavior during a test situation. Further, a quantitative researcher might obtain a series of specific observations before considering the theoretical bases for the study. An inductive approach is not exclusive to qualitative research.

Because of their training and preferences, some researchers might consider themselves to be primarily qualitative researchers. Such persons would tend to approach most problems from a qualitative perspective. As we noted, however, qualitative and quantitative research are not exclusive approaches, and sometimes the decision to use a qualitative or quantitative approach is based on the nature of the problem rather than on researcher preferences (Gillham, 2000; Patten, 2007). Some problems might be inherently suited to a qualitative approach. If very little is known about a problem, if recruiting participants requires special care, if a problem is best understood through the viewpoint of an "insider," or if a problem is best approached through long-term interaction and observation, researchers might favor a qualitative approach (Gillham, 2000; Patten, 2007).

One of the roles of a research design is to assure that the results of a study accurately reflect the actual or real situation. Damico and Simmons-Mackie (2003, p. 133) noted that "interpretive adequacy" is the goal of qualitative research. One might think of interpretative adequacy as "describing and explaining" an experience in a way that reflects the participants' understanding of it and also captures its meaning to society in general (Damico & Simmons-Mackie, 2003). Qualitative researchers might choose one of several approaches when designing a study or even combine approaches (Trochim & Donnelly, 2007). In the following sections, we briefly describe several of these approaches to illustrate the options available for qualitative studies.

Ethnography

Ethnographic research emerged from the field of anthropology and encompasses several methods of studying events or behaviors within their cultural context (Berg, 2001; Damico & Simmons-Mackie, 2003). Two concepts closely tied to ethnography are participant observation and field research (Trochim & Donnelly, 2007). Researchers using ethnographic methods spend considerable time in the situation or culture they are studying. That is, they spend time "in the field" initially to gain acceptance as a participant and eventually to gather information from persons within the culture. The methods used in participant observation include writing down detailed field notes, interviewing persons from the culture, and collecting cultural artifacts (Gillham, 2000; Miller, Hengst, & Wang, 2003).

Historically, anthropologists traveled to a remote geographic location to study a native culture. However, in contemporary applications of ethnographic methods, the notion of culture has a broader definition and might include the culture of a classroom, of a particular organization, of an event, and so forth. One thing that sets scientific inquiry apart is its systematic nature. Miller, Hengst, and Wang (2003) noted that researchers using ethnographic methods achieve scientific rigor through the number and extent of their observations, the detailed way they record or describe their observations, repeated review of their data, and ongoing revision of interpretations or conclusions.

Grounded Theory

Qualitative researchers using a grounded theory approach have the goal of developing conceptual or theoretical models to account for observed behaviors, events, situations, and so forth. Trochim and Donnelly (2007, p. 182) described the product of grounded theory research as " . . . an extremely well-considered explanation for some phenomenon of interest—the grounded theory." The data obtained to develop such a theory are similar to that collected in an ethnographic approach. Thus, a researcher will conduct interviews, make observations in the field, and collect documents for analysis. However, grounded theory methods are more formally structured than most other qualitative research approaches; for that reason, grounded theory is often an attractive approach for persons who are beginning researchers (Henwood & Pidgeon, 2003).

Grounded theory research could be described as a recurring process of collecting data, examining and coding data, and generating theoretical concepts or categories. According to Henwood and Pidgeon (2003), the initial step after a round of data collection is to examine the data and generate codes that emerge from the data rather than from preexisting expectations. This process is sometimes called *open coding* and requires researchers to be flexible in their thinking and open to new ideas or insights evoked by the data. After developing this initial set of codes, researchers compare codes across different individuals, situations, and types of data (e.g., observation notes, interview transcripts) to identify similarities and differences (Henwood & Pidgeon, 2003).

The first phase of data collection, coding, and comparison is the foundation for additional data collection and coding. Researchers need to reexamine and revise concepts based on the new data. As concepts and theoretical notions emerge, additional data collection is more focused and designed to test these initial ideas. While coding their data, researchers begin the writing process by noting concepts that emerged and how these concepts relate to ideas from the existing literature (Henwood & Pidgeon, 2003). Are the emerging concepts similar or different and in what ways? According to Henwood and Pidgeon, researchers engage in data collection and coding until it is no longer productive and no new "relevant insights" emerge (p. 136). In the final phases of a grounded theory study, researchers begin focusing on developing a theory or explanation that fits the data. As part of this process, they reexamine how they organized data into categories, identify the "core categories" in the data, and consider how these categories might fit into broader concepts or models (p. 136). Ultimately, the adequacy of a grounded theory approach depends on how successful researchers were in generating a theory that fits their specific observations and also provides explanatory power.

Case Study

As noted previously, case study researchers might collect quantitative data, qualitative data, or a mixture of both (Hancock & Algozzine, 2006). When approached from a qualitative perspective, case study research methods have considerable overlap with the methods of ethnography and grounded theory. Researchers spend time observing the case, conducting interviews, and reviewing various kinds of documents. What distinguishes case study research is the focus on an entity such as a person, event, family, or institution (Berg, 2001; Damico & Simmons-Mackie, 2003). When designing a case study, researchers consider how broadly they want to investigate the case. Sometimes the scope of a study is all-inclusive, researchers attempt to gather data from as many sources as possible, and they try to understand the influences that determine how the case functions within society (Berg, 2001). At other times, a case study is highly focused; researchers gather data only at a particular time, or they gather data regarding one of the case's many roles. When conducting a focused case study, researchers are trying to understand the influences that determined the case's actions and motivations at a particular time or when performing a particular role (Berg, 2001).

Berg (2001) noted that researchers have different goals when conducting case study research. In an *intrinsic* case study, the researchers' goal is to understand the particular entity they are studying, rather than to understand a larger context such as a culture or the organization of social behavior. In an *instrumental* case study,

researchers identify a case that represents a phenomenon they want to study. They conduct a thorough investigation of this case by gathering data through various methods such as observation, multiple interviews, and examination of documents. The researchers' aim is to discover answers to questions of general interest in their field of study, rather than to gain insight into the behaviors and motivations of the individual case. Finally, in a *collective* case study, researchers identify several instrumental cases and gather data from all of them. A more extensive set of data should enhance researchers' ability to draw conclusions or gain insights that will generalize to other, similar entities (Berg, 2001).

Phenomenology

The goal of researchers who adopt a *phenomenology* approach is to study a phenomenon or situation from the viewpoint of participants (Trochim & Donnelly, 2007). Researchers try to discover what participants perceive, how they interpret a situation, and what meanings they assign to events. Giorgi and Giorgi (2003) described an adaptation of phenomenology for scientific investigation in the field of psychology. In this version of phenomenology, researchers begin by obtaining "descriptions of experiences" from participants, often through interviews (Giorgi & Giorgi, 2003, p. 247). In the next phase of the study, researchers read transcriptions of the interviews to gain an overall impression of the content, and then to divide the transcript into "psychological meaning units" (Giorgi & Giorgi, 2003, p. 254). Giorgi and Giorgi noted that researchers typically notice a change or transition in meaning as they read the linear interview transcripts. Once researchers have a transcript that is divided into a series of meaning units, the next step is to translate these meaning units into a few words that capture the "psychological meaning lived by P [the participant]" (Giorgi & Giorgi, 2003, p. 254). Some examples of these interpretations include "feelings of emotional ambivalence" and "feelings of unsafety" (Giorgi & Giorgi, 2003, p. 256).

In phenomenology researchers use a mental process, "free imaginative variation," to discern the meaning that underlies a section of the interview transcript (Giorgi & Giorgi, 2003, p. 246). This is a process of mental manipulation in which the researcher imagines variations of the situation or phenomenon. For example, researchers might imagine a situation with different participants, taking place in a different location, or with different conversational content. Researchers focus on those imagined variations that change the sense of the situation, because those variations point to the psychological meaning for the participants.[2] Although researchers demonstrate the association between statements from the interview transcript and their psychological interpretations, researchers often use words that were not part of the participants' description of the situation to highlight the meaning. As a way of avoiding a priori assumptions from existing theories, researchers should express psychological meaning in the everyday language of participants rather than in terminology taken from the professional literature. In the final phase, researchers describe the structure of an experience, focusing on those meanings that were constant across " . . . a series of experiences of the same type" (Giorgi & Giorgi, 2003, p. 258).

Quantitative research approaches are far more common in the field of communi-cation sciences and disorders than qualitative approaches. However, several good examples are available in recent articles on uses of feedback in treatment of persons with aphasia (Simmons-Mackie, Damico, & Damico, 1999), communication in persons with multiple sclerosis (Yorkston, Klasner, & Swanson, 2001), mothers of children with fragile X syndrome (Brady, Skinner, Roberts, & Hennon, 2006), how mothers who immi-grated from Mexico viewed their children's communication disorders and speech-language services (Kummerer, Lopez-Reyna, & Hughes, 2007), the role of school-based speech-language pathologists in providing language services (Ukrainetz & Fresquez, 2003), and analysis of discourse in therapy for a child who stuttered (Leahy, 2004).

Scientific Rigor in Qualitative Research

One of the functions of a research design is to establish the validity or credibility of the researchers' findings. In qualitative approaches, researchers might not use the term validity, but they do use other similar terms, such as trustworthy, plausible, or credible (Golafshani, 2003; Patten, 2007). Thus, when designing a qualitative study, researchers include procedures to demon-strate that their findings accurately portray the actual phenomenon or accurately inter-pret participants' experiences.

Some common issues that qualitative researchers need to address include re-searcher bias, descriptive adequacy, and interpretive adequacy. All persons have pre-vious experiences, knowledge, and points

---

[2]For a more concrete description of a phenomenological approach, you might consider reading Giorgi and Giorgi (2003, pp. 246–247). The authors used the example of imagining differences in a tangible object, a cup, to illustrate the process of free imaginative variation.

of view that predispose them to act and to interpret new experiences in certain ways. In other words, all persons have sources of bias that influence their actions and thoughts. When researchers allow their previous experiences, knowledge, and points of view to influence their observation and interpretation of a phenomenon, the researcher is exhibiting *researcher bias*. In an extreme form, researchers might be selective in what they see, hear, and record due to this bias. The issue of researcher bias is crucial for qualitative approaches because the findings depend on the researchers' observations, field notes, interview questions, and interpretations. However, eliminating the sources of bias, that is the researchers' previous experiences, knowledge, and points of view, is unrealistic. Instead, qualitative researchers take steps to demonstrate that their data and interpretations were not unduly influenced by these preexisting influences.

One strategy for minimizing bias is *reflexivity*. Researchers consider their previous experiences and beliefs associated with the topic of the study and reflect on how these experiences and beliefs might have influenced how they approached the research question, data collection, and interpretation (Jaye, 2002). Researchers sometimes overtly discuss their potential biases in their research notes or report. Another strategy researchers might use to address potential biases is *negative case sampling*. Given an awareness of how their prior experiences and beliefs could influence their findings, researchers might test their conclusions by a deliberate attempt to find instances in their data, or perhaps to collect new data, that are at odds with these conclusions (Bowen, 2005). Another strategy to address researcher bias is to use a triangulation strategy. In *researcher triangulation*, more than one person participates in developing the research question, collecting data,

and analyzing and interpreting the findings (Patten, 2007). If researchers with diverse backgrounds arrive at the same interpretations of the findings, the conclusions from the study are stronger.

To demonstrate *descriptive adequacy*, researchers need to show that they provided an accurate factual account of the events they observed and experiences participants reported. In addition, researchers try to demonstrate that they collected sufficient data to provide meaningful insights into the phenomenon under study. One strategy researchers use to enhance their descriptive adequacy is *prolonged engagement* in the field (Creswell & Miller, 2000). By spending more time in the field, researchers build greater rapport with participants, are more likely to observe significant events, and have opportunities to observe phenomena repeatedly. Researchers also use various forms of triangulation to increase descriptive adequacy. In *methods triangulation*, a researcher uses several different strategies to collect data, such as observation in the field, interview of participants, and review of documents (Patten, 2007); and in *data triangulation*, a researcher collects data from several different participants using a similar strategy. For example, the researcher could interview a person with a communication disorder, interview one or more of his peers, interview family members, and perhaps interview an employer or teacher. A final strategy researchers might employ is *thick description*. A thick description is a highly detailed, specific description of a phenomenon. A researcher could prepare a factual account of a situation or event without achieving the level of a thick description. What sets a thick description apart is how thoroughly the researcher describes an event. For example, if researchers were describing an interaction between a parent and child, they would include details about

s, what artifacts are pres-
tails about the behaviors of

etive adequacy of qualita-
depends on how well the
researchers captured and conveyed the meaning of an experience. When qualitative researchers focus on what an experience means to the participants, *participant feedback* is the primary strategy for establishing interpretive adequacy. The researchers might ask participants to read a factual description or an interpretation of an event, conversation, series of behaviors, and so forth. Then, the participants provide their views on the accuracy of the description or interpretation (Creswell & Miller, 2000).

Qualitative researchers might or might not use the term validity when referring to how well their findings represent an actual phenomenon. However, they almost always would include some of the above strategies, or similar ones, to demonstrate that their research was credible and trustworthy.

Summary

For some research questions, the best approach is to study an existing situation or phenomenon. Nonexperimental research, like experimental research, is a systematic form of inquiry with the goal of finding answers to relevant questions. However, experimental research involves deliberate manipulation of the variable under investigation, and nonexperimental research involves studying a variable or difference that already is present. One might think of nonexperimental research as studying differences that are naturally occurring, and experimental research as studying differences planned and created by the researchers. Researchers have many methods for inves-

tigating problems in a nonexperimental way. In the field of communication sciences and disorders, examples of nonexperimental research include surveys, case studies, prevalence studies, correlation and prediction studies, group comparisons, and causal-comparative studies. Although nonexperimental research approaches involve studying naturally occurring phenomena, they still include the features of systematic inquiry, such as a well-thought-out question, and a plan for collecting and analyzing data to answer that question.

Qualitative research encompasses a number of research approaches such as case studies, ethnography, grounded theory, and phenomenology. Qualitative researchers often gather data in the natural context of their participants' everyday lives, using methods such as observation in the field, collection and analysis of documents, and interviews. Usually researchers collect, analyze, and report verbal data in the form of oral or written statements and detailed descriptions. Another characteristic is that researchers usually rely on inductive reasoning, beginning with specific forms of information, and generating concepts and theories that fit that data. To enhance the credibility of their findings, qualitative researchers collect an extensive amount of data, often recruit more than one participant, use several data collection strategies, and check their observations and interpretations with other researchers as well as with the participants.

Review Questions

1. What is the primary difference between experimental and nonexperimental research designs?

2. Match the type of nonexperimental study with its description.

_____ Survey research
_____ Correlation study
_____ Group comparison
_____ Case study

a. Compare persons with and without communication disorders
b. Study a single person, situation, or organization
c. Obtain participants' responses to questions
d. Determine the relationship between two variables

3. Are case studies an example of qualitative or quantitative research? Explain your answer.

4. Do researchers conduct correlation studies to establish a cause and effect relationship between two variables?

5. Explain how researchers test their participants when conducting a prediction study.

6. What kind of study is the best alternative for identifying potential cause and effect relationships when conducting a true experiment is not practical?

7. Identify the characteristics of qualitative research. Choose all that apply.
a. Researchers using this approach rely on inductive reasoning.
b. Researchers often use this research approach when very little is known about a topic.
c. This research method usually yields a statistical report of results.

d. The results might include quotes from the participants' statements.
e. The researcher usually spends only a short time with each participant.

8. Which of the following research questions is most appropriate for a quantitative approach? Which is most appropriate for a qualitative approach? Explain your answers.
a. What are the differences between the school interactions, both with peers and teachers, of fifth-grade students with communication disorders and fifth-grade students with typical communication?
b. To what extent does parent education level predict the interaction skills of parents of 1-year-old infants with a history of very low birth weight and parents of 1-year-old infants with normal birth weight?

9. Which of the following are nonexperimental research approaches? Select all that apply.
a. randomly assigning participants to treatment and control groups
b. correlation study comparing scores on two tests
c. comparing children with communication disorders to age-matched peers
d. A-B-A-B single subject design
e. survey of a random sample of speech-language pathologists

10. What "threat" to credibility or validity might be occurring in the following scenario? A qualitative researcher was interested in studying how children

with specific language impairment (SLI) communicated with their classroom teachers. The researcher believed that SLI would interfere with effective classroom communication. The researcher only wrote down instances in which communication breakdowns occurred between the children and their teachers.

11. List two strategies qualitative researchers use to address the issue of researcher bias.

12. How do qualitative researchers assure that they have accurately portrayed the *meaning* of their participants' actions, statements, and beliefs?

Learning Activities

1. To learn more about one of nonexperimental research approaches covered in this chapter, read studies that exemplify that approach.

Survey Research

Allen, M. S., Pettit, J. M., & Sherblom, J. C. (1991). Management of vocal nodules: A regional survey of otolaryngologists and speech-language pathologists. *Journal of Speech and Hearing Research*, *34*, 229–235.

Hoffman, J. M., Yorkston, K. M., Shumway-Cook, A., Ciol, M. A., Dudgeon, B. J., & Chan, L. (2005). Effect of communication disability on satisfaction with health care: A survey of Medicare beneficiaries. *American Journal of Speech-Language Pathology*, *14*, 221–228.

Roseberry-McKibbin, C., Brice, A., & O'Hanlon, L. (2005). Serving English language learners in public school settings: A national survey. *Language, Speech, and Hearing Services and Schools*, *36*, 48–61.

Case Study

Craig, H. K., & Telfor, A. S. (2005). Hyperlexia and autism spectrum disorder: A case study of scaffolding language growth over time. *Topics in Language Disorders*, *25*, 364–324.

Worth, S., & Reynolds, S. (2008). The assessment and identification of language impairment in Asperger's syndrome: A case study. *Child Language Teaching and Therapy*, *24*, 55–71.

Correlational Research

Rabinowitz, P. M., Galusha, D., Dixon-Ernst, C., Slade, M. D., & Cullen, M. R. (2007). Do ambient noise exposure levels predict hearing loss in a modern industrial cohort? *Occupational and Environmental Medicine*, *64*(10), 53–59.

Rescorla, L., Rattner, N. B., Jusczyk, P., & Jusczyk, A. M. (2005). Concurrent validity of the language development survey: Associations with the MacArthur-Bates communicative development inventories: Words and sentences. *American Journal of Speech-Language Pathology*, *14*(2), 156–163.

Wheeler, K. M., Collins, S. P., & Sapienza, C. M. (2006). The relationship between VHI scores and specific acoustic measures of mildly disordered voice production. *Journal of Voice*, *20*(2), 308–317.

Group Comparison

Archibald, L. M. D., & Gathercole, S. E. (2006). Visuospatial immediate memory in specific language impairment. *Journal of Speech, Language, and Hearing Research*, *49*, 265–277.

Bajaj, A. (2007). Analysis of oral narratives of children who stutter and their fluent peers: Kindergarten through second grade. *Clinical Linguistics & Phonetics*, *21*(3), 227–245.

Hicks, C. B. & Tharpe, A. M. (2002). Listening effort and fatigue in school-age children with and without hearing loss. *Journal of Speech, Language, and Hearing Research, 45*, 573–584.

Moeller, M. P., Hoover, B., Putnam, C., Arbataitis, K., Bohnenkamp, G., Petersen, B., et al. (2007). Vocalizations of infants with hearing loss compared with infants with normal hearing. Part I: Phonetic development. *Ear and Hearing, 28,* 605–627.

Causal-Comparative Study

Aram, D. M., Hack, M., Hawkins, S., Weissman, B. M., & Borawski-Clark, E. (1991). Very-low-birthweight children and speech and language development. *Journal of Speech and Hearing Research, 34,* 1169–1179.

Kilbride, H. W., Thorstad, K., & Daily, D. K. (2004). Preschool outcome of less than 801-gram preterm infants compared with full-term siblings. *Pediatrics, 113,* 742–747.

Shriberg, L. D., Flipsen, P., Jr., Thielke, H., Kwiatkowski, J., Kertoy, M. K., Katcher, M. L., et al. (2000). Risk for speech disorder associated with early recurrent otitis media with effusion: Two retrospective studies. *Journal of Speech, Language, and Hearing Research, 43,* 79–99.

Qualitative Research

Brady, N., Skinner, D., Roberts, J., & Hennon, E. (2006). Communication in young children with fragile X syndrome: A qualitative study of mothers' perspectives. *American Journal of Speech-Language Pathology, 15,* 353–364.

Kummerer, S. E., Lopez-Reyna, N. A., & Hughes, M. R. (2007). Mexican immigrant mothers' perceptions of their children's communication disabilities, emergent literacy development, and speech-language therapy program. *American Journal of Speech-Language Pathology, 16,* 271–282.

Simmons-Mackie, N., Damico, J. S., & Damico, H. L. (1999). A qualitative study of feedback in aphasia treatment. *American Journal of Speech-Language Pathology, 8,* 218–230.

Yorkston, K. M., Klasner, E. R., & Swanson, K. M. (2001). Communication in context: A qualitative study of the experiences of individuals with multiple sclerosis. *American Journal of Speech-Language Pathology, 10,* 126–137.

2. Select one of the following hypothetical research scenarios. Decide what research approach you would use. Provide some examples of the issues you need to consider in planning such a study.

   a. A graduate student wants to investigate the effects of communication disorders on the daily activities and participation patterns of persons with speech, language, or hearing disorders. Help the student develop a more detailed research question and research design. What research approach(es) should this student consider?

   b. A school-based speech-language pathologist (SLP) developed a procedure called *Rapid Spontaneous Speech Analysis*, which is a relatively quick way to assess preschool and school-aged children's spontaneous conversation. This SLP wants to conduct a study to determine if this new procedure is a valid measure of expressive language skills. Help the SLP develop a more detailed research question and research design. What research approach(es) should this SLP consider?

References

Allen, M. S., Pettit, J. M., & Sherblom, J. C. (1991). Management of vocal nodules: A regional survey of otolaryngologists and speech-language pathologists. *Journal of Speech and Hearing Research, 34,* 229–235.

American Academy of Audiology. (2006). *Compensations & benefits survey.* Retrieved January 8, 2008, from http://www.audiology.org/membership/benefits/compsurvey/default.htm?PF=1

American Speech-Language-Hearing Association. (2006a). *Audiology surveys.* Retrieved January 11, 2008, from http://www.asha.org/members/aud/Audsur.htm

American Speech-Language-Hearing Association. (2006b). *2006 schools survey reports.* Retrieved January 11, 2008, from http://www.asha.org/members/slp/schools/resources/2006Schools survey

American Speech-Language-Hearing Association. (2007). *2007 SLP healthcare survey reports.* Retrieved January 11, 2008, from http://www.asha.org/about/membership-certification/member-data/HealthcareSurvey07.htm

Aram, D. M., Hack, M., Hawkins, S., Weissman, B. M., & Borawski-Clark, E. (1991). Very-low-birthweight children and speech and language development. *Journal of Speech and Hearing Research, 34,* 1169–1179.

Archibald, L. M. D., & Gathercole, S. E. (2006). Visuospatial immediate memory in specific language impairment. *Journal of Speech, Language, and Hearing Research, 49,* 265–277.

Bajaj, A. (2007). Analysis of oral narratives of children who stutter and their fluent peers: Kindergarten through second grade. *Clinical Linguistics & Phonetics, 21*(3), 227–245.

Berg, B. L. (2001). *Qualitative research methods for the social sciences* (4th ed.). Boston: Allyn & Bacon.

Blischak, D. M. (1995). Thomas the writer: Case study of a child with severe physical, speech, and visual impairments. *Language, Speech, and Hearing Services in Schools, 26,* 11–20.

Bowen, G. A. (2005). Preparing a qualitative research-based dissertation: Lessons learned [Electronic version]. *The Qualitative Report, 10,* 208–222.

Brady, N., Skinner, D., Roberts, J., & Hennon, E. (2006). Communication in young children with fragile X syndrome: A qualitative study of mothers' perspectives. *American Journal of Speech-Language Pathology, 15,* 353–364.

Clark, D. G., Charuvastra, A., Miller, B. L., Shapira, J. S., & Mendez, M. F. (2005). Fluent versus nonfluent primary progressive aphasia: A comparison of clinical and functional neuroimaging features. *Brain and Language, 94,* 54–60.

Craig, H. K., & Telfor, A. S. (2005). Hyperlexia and autism spectrum disorder: A case study of scaffolding language growth over time. *Topics in Language Disorders, 25,* 364–324.

Creswell, J. W., & Miller, D. L. (2000). Determining validity in qualitative inquiry [Electronic version]. *Theory into Practice: Getting Good Qualitative Data to Improve Educational Practice, 39*(3), 124–130.

Damico, J. S., & Simmons-Mackie, N. N. (2003). Qualitative research and speech-language pathology: A tutorial for the clinical realm. *American Journal of Speech-Language Pathology, 12,* 131–143.

Estes, K. G., Evans, J. L., & Else-Quest, N. M. (2007). Differences in the nonword repetition performance of children with and without specific language impairment: A meta-analysis. *Journal of Speech, Language, and Hearing Research, 50,* 177–195.

Foster-Cohen, S., Edgin, J. O., Champion, P. R., & Woodward, L. J. (2007). Early delayed language development in very preterm infants: Evidence from the MacArthur-Bates CDI. *Journal of Child Language, 34,* 655–675.

Fowler, C. G., Kile, J. E., & Hecox, K. E. (2001). Electrical status epilepticus in slow wave sleep: Prospective case study of a cortical hearing impairment. *Journal of the American Academy of Audiology, 12*(4), 174–182.

Fridriksson, J., Nettles, C., Davis, M., Morrow, L., & Montgomery, A. (2006). Functional communication and executive function in aphasia. *Clinical Linguistics & Phonetics, 20*(6), 401–410.

Gillham, B. (2000). *Case study research methods.* London: Continuum.

Giorgi, A. P., & Giorgi, B. M. (2003). The descriptive phenomenological psychological method. In P. M. Camic, J. E. Rhodes, & L. Yardley (Eds.), *Qualitative research in psychology: Expanding perspectives in methodology and design* (pp. 243–259). Washington, DC: American Psychological Association.

Golafshani, N. (2003). Understanding reliability and validity in qualitative research [Electronic version]. *The Qualitative Report, 8,* 597–607.

Gordon-Salant, S., Fitzgibbons, P. J., & Friedman, S. A. (2007). Recognition of time-compressed and natural speech with selective temporal enhancements by young and elderly listeners. *Journal of Speech, Language, and Hearing Research, 50,* 1181–1193.

Goulandris, N. K., Snowling, M. J., & Walker, I. (2000). Is dyslexia a form of specific language impairment? A comparison of dyslexia and language impaired children as adolescents. *Annals of Dyslexia, 50,* 103–120.

Hancock, D. R., & Algozzine, B. (2006). *Doing case study research: A practical guide for beginning researchers.* New York: Teacher's College Press.

Henwood, K., & Pidgeon, N. (2003). Grounded theory in psychological research. In P. M. Camic, J. E. Rhodes, & L. Yardley (Eds.), *Qualitative research in psychology: Expanding perspectives in methodology and design* (pp. 131–155). Washington, DC: American Psychological Association.

Hicks, C. B ., & Tharpe, A. M. (2002). Listening effort and fatigue in school-age children with and without hearing loss. *Journal of Speech, Language, and Hearing Research, 45,* 573–584.

Hoffman, J. M., Yorkston, K. M., Shumway-Cook, A., Ciol, M. A., Dudgeon, B. J., & Chan, L. (2005). Effect of communication disability on satisfaction with health care: A survey of Medicare beneficiaries. *American Journal of Speech-Language Pathology, 14,* 221–228.

Hogan, T. P., Catts, H. W., & Little, T. D. (2005). The relationship between phonological awareness and reading: Implications for the assessment of phonological awareness. *Language, Speech, and Hearing Services in Schools, 36*(4), 385–393.

Horga, D., & Liker, M. (2006). Voice and pronunciation of cochlear implant speakers. *Clinical Linguistics & Phonetics, 20,* 211–217.

Ingles, J. L., Fisk, J. D., Passmore, M., & Darvesh, S. (2007). Progressive anomia without semantic or phonological impairment. *Cortex, 43*(4), 558–564.

Jaye, C. (2002). Doing qualitative research in general practice: Methodological utility and engagement [Electronic version]. *Family Practice, 19,* 557–562.

Kilbride, H. W., Thorstad, K., & Daily, D. K. (2004). Preschool outcome of less than 801-gram preterm infants compared with full-term siblings. *Pediatrics, 113,* 742–747.

Kummerer, S. E., Lopez-Reyna, N. A., & Hughes, M. R. (2007). Mexican immigrant mothers' perceptions of their children's communication disabilities, emergent literacy development, and speech-language therapy program. *American Journal of Speech-Language Pathology, 16,* 271–282.

Larney, R. (2002). The relationship between early language delay and later difficulties in literacy. *Early Child Development and Care, 172*(2), 182–193.

Leahy, M. M. (2004). Therapy talk analyzing therapeutic discourse. *Language, Speech, and Hearing Services in Schools, 35,* 70–81.

Mendez, M. F., Clark, D. G., Shapira, J. S., & Cummings, J. L. (2003). Speech and language in progressive nonfluent aphasia compared with early Alzheimer's disease. *Neurology, 61,* 1108–1113.

Miller, P. J., Hengst, J. A., & Wang, S.-H. (2003). Ethnographic methods: Applications from developmental cultural psychology. In P. M. Camic, J. E. Rhodes, & L. Yardley (Eds.), *Qualitative research in psychology: Expanding perspectives in methodology and design* (pp. 219–242). Washington, DC: American Psychological Association.

Moeller, M. P., Hoover, B., Putnam, C., Arbataitis, K., Bohnenkamp, G., Petersen, B., et al. (2007). Vocalizations of infants with hearing loss compared with infants with normal hearing. Part I: Phonetic development. *Ear and Hearing, 28,* 605–627.

Newman, R. S., & Ratner, N. B. (2007). The role of selected lexical factors on confrontation naming accuracy, speed, and fluency in adults who do and do not stutter. *Journal of Speech, Language, and Hearing Disorders, 50*, 196-213.

Pankratz, M. E., Plante, E., Vance, R., & Insalaco, D. M. (2007). The diagnostic and predictive validity of the Renfrew Bus Story. *Language, Speech, and Hearing Services in Schools, 38*, 390-399.

Patten, M. L. (2007). *Understanding research methods: An overview of the essentials* (6th ed.). Glendale, CA: Pyrczak.

Rabinowitz, P. M., Galusha, D., Dixon-Ernst, C., Slade, M. D., & Cullen, M. R. (2007). Do ambient noise exposure levels predict hearing loss in a modern industrial cohort? *Occupational and Environmental Medicine, 64*(10), 53-59.

Reilly, W., Walk, M., Bavin, E. L., Prior, M., Williams, J., Bretherton, L., et al. (2007). Predicting language at 2 years of age. A prospective community study [Electronic version]. *Pediatrics, 120*(6), e1441-1449.

Rescorla, L., Rattner, N. B., Jusczyk, P., & Jusczyk, A. M. (2005). Concurrent validity of the language development survey: Associations with the MacArthur-Bates communicative development inventories: Words and sentences. *American Journal of Speech-Language Pathology, 14*(2), 156-163.

Roberts, J. E., Rosenfeld, R. M., & Zeisel, S. A. (2004). Otitis media and speech and language: A meta-analysis of prospective studies [Electronic version]. *Pediatrics, 113*, e238-248.

Roseberry-McKibbin, C., Brice, A., & O'Hanlon, L. (2005). Serving English language learners in public school settings: A national survey. *Language, Speech, and Hearing Services and Schools, 36*, 48-61.

Roy, N., Merrill, R. M., Thibeault, S., Gray, S. D., & Smith, E. M. (2004). Voice disorders in teachers and the general population: Effects on work performance, attendance, and future career choices. *Journal of Speech, Language, and Hearing Research, 47*, 542-551.

Saygin, A. P., Wilson, S. M., Dronkers, N. F., & Bates, E. (2004). Action comprehension in aphasia: Linguistic and non-linguistic deficits and their lesion correlates. *Neuropsychologia, 42*, 1788-1804.

Schwartz, H., & Drager, K. D. R. (2008). Training and knowledge in autism among speech-language pathologists: A survey. *Language, Speech, and Hearing Services and Schools, 39*, 66-77.

Shriberg, L. D., Flipsen, P., Jr., Thielke, H., Kwiatkowski, J., Kertoy, M. K., Katcher, M. L., et al. (2000). Risk for speech disorder associated with early recurrent otitis media with effusion: Two retrospective studies. *Journal of Speech, Language, and Hearing Research, 43*, 79-99.

Shriberg, L. D., Friel-Patti, S., Flipsen, P., Jr., & Brown, R. L. (2000). Otitis media, fluctuant hearing loss, and speech-language outcomes: A preliminary structural equation model. *Journal of Speech, Language, and Hearing Research, 43*, 100-120.

Simmons-Mackie, N., Damico, J. S., & Damico, H. L. (1999). A qualitative study of feedback in aphasia treatment. *American Journal of Speech-Language Pathology, 8*, 218-230.

Takayanagi, S., Dirks, D. D., & Moshfegh, A. (2002). Lexical and talker effects on word recognition among native and non-native listeners with normal and impaired hearing. *Journal of Speech, Language, and Hearing Research, 45*, 585-597.

Tharpe, A. M., Fino-Szumski, M. S., & Bess, F. H. (2001). Survey of hearing aid fitting practices for children with multiple impairments. *American Journal of Audiology, 10*, 32-40.

Trochim, W. M. K., & Donnelly, J. P. (2007). *The research methods knowledge base* (3rd ed.). Mason, OH: Thomson Custom.

Ukrainetz, T. A., & Fresquez, E. F. (2003). What isn't language? A qualitative study of the role of the school speech-language pathologist. *Language, Speech, and Hearing Services in Schools, 34*, 284-298.

Wheeler, K. M., Collins, S. P., & Sapienza, C. M. (2006). The relationship between VHI scores and specific acoustic measures of mildly disordered voice production. *Journal of Voice, 20*(2), 308-317.

Wetherell, D., Botting, N., & Conti-Ramsden, G. (2007). Narrative in adolescent specific language impairment (SLI): A comparison with peers across two different narrative genres. *International Journal of Language and Communication Disorders, 42,* 583–605.

Worth, S., & Reynolds, S. (2008). The assessment and identification of language impairment in Asperger's syndrome: A case study. *Child Language Teaching and Therapy, 24,* 55–71.

Writing Center at Colorado State University. (2008). *Overview: Survey research.* Retrieved January 11, 2008, from http://writing.colo state.edu/guides/research/survey/

Yorkston, K. M., Klasner, E. R., & Swanson, K. M. (2001). Communication in context: A qualitative study of the experiences of individuals with multiple sclerosis. *American Journal of Speech-Language Pathology, 10,* 126–137.

CHAPTER 6

Experimental Research and Levels of Evidence

An important step in conducting empirical research is to develop a plan or design for making observations and collecting data. The particular features of this design will depend on the nature of the problem you are investigating. One of the initial decisions is whether to design a study that uses experimental or nonexperimental procedures. For example, do you need to change a situation in some way, perhaps by providing an experimental treatment, to answer your question? Or can you answer your question simply by making observations and measurements of existing phenomena? If researchers intend to obtain evidence to support a cause and effect relationship, an experimental research design is nearly always the best approach[1] (Trochim & Donnelly, 2007). In an *experimental research design*, researchers identify one or more factors that they will manipulate or control during the experiment (Patten, 2007). The variables that researchers manipulate are called *independent variables*. Researchers also identify one or more ways that they will measure the outcomes of the experiment. That is, they measure the effects of their experimental manipulation on the participants' behavior. These outcome measures are called *dependent variables*. The point of experimental research is to establish that the experimental manipulation is the reason for any differences observed in the participants' performance on the outcome measures.

Audiologists and speech-language pathologists usually think of the term *treatment* as referring to the actions we take to improve our clients' speech, language, and/or hearing. However, researchers use the term treatment in a broader sense. The term treatment in experimental research refers to the conditions you manipulate or the independent variable(s). Certainly, the experimental manipulation might be a comparison of two treatments in the therapeutic sense. That is, the researcher might be interested in which of two treatments leads to the most improvement at the end of a study. However, the experimental manipulation might

---

[1]In Chapter 4 we discussed instances when researchers would be interested in cause and effect relationships, such as the cause of a particular speech, language, or hearing disorder, but experimental manipulation of the causal variable would be inappropriate. Research in which persons are deliberately exposed to a variable that could cause a communication disorder would be unethical.

be something that does not have a lasting therapeutic effect. For example, researchers might study persons with normal communication abilities to determine how two different presentation modes affect their performance on a task. This experimental manipulation would not produce a lasting improvement in the participants' abilities but would still be considered a "treatment" effect when discussing the results of such a study.

Researchers make a number of decisions in planning an experimental study. They decide on the different treatments or experiences participants will receive during the study and how to measure the outcomes associated with those different treatments. In addition, they make decisions about recruiting participants and when to obtain outcome measures. The procedures for recruiting and selecting participants are covered in another chapter. However, when to obtain outcome measures is a characteristic of the research designs we cover in this chapter. In some research approaches, participants are tested only once at the end of a study. In other approaches, they might be tested both at the beginning and at the end of the study or even a couple of times after the end of the study.

An additional decision researchers make during the planning phase relates to the number of different treatments they will compare. When discussing the number of treatments, researchers sometimes use a phrase such as *levels of the independent variable* or *levels of treatment*. Previously, we considered examples in which researchers compared two different treatments or manipulations. However, researchers could design a study in which they compared three or more different treatments, depending on what comparisons were logical as well as practical. What is logical depends on the nature of the problem the researchers are investigating and on the answers available from previous research. What is practical depends primarily on the number of participants you can recruit for the study. For example, some types of communication disorders have a relatively low prevalence and recruiting enough participants to divide into even two treatment groups could be a challenge.

In the following sections on research design, we make a distinction between *true experimental designs* (i.e., experimental research designs) and *quasi-experimental designs*. Both experimental and quasi-experimental research designs incorporate one feature—researcher manipulation of a variable. The researcher creates different conditions or experiences for the participants by manipulating one or more factors during the study (Patten, 2007; Trochim & Donnelly, 2007). Only a true experimental design incorporates the second feature of random assignment of participants to different experimental groups. Generally speaking, a study that incorporates both features, experimental manipulation and random assignment, provides stronger evidence than a quasi-experimental study. Thus, in the discussion that follows, those research designs that are true experimental designs provide a stronger or higher level of evidence than those that are classified as quasi-experimental.

Experimental Research Designs

In this section we describe several experimental research designs. To illustrate each of the designs, we will use a common system of notation to represent the various steps in the research design (e.g., Patten, 2007; Trochim & Donnelly, 2007). For example, one of the things researchers must do is observe and obtain measures of their participants' behavior. In the notation system, the letter O represents an observation and measurement step. Another step in experimental research is to implement a treatment or manipulation of some variable. The letter X represents application of the experimental treatment. Finally, in a true experimental design, the participants are randomly assigned to the various treatment groups at the beginning of the study. The letter R represents the step of random assignment to groups.

Posttest-Only Designs

The most basic example of a true experimental design is a *posttest-only randomized control group design* (Patten, 2007; Trochim & Donnelly, 2007). In this design, the researchers randomly assign participants to different treatment groups, implement the different treatments, and then observe and measure their participants' behavior. This design is considered a posttest-only design because the participants are tested only after they complete the treatment step. The notation for this type of design is as follows:

Example 1

Posttest-Only Randomized Control Group

| R | X | O |
| R | | O |

In this design, the two rows beginning with R illustrate random assignment of participants to two different groups. The sequence R X O means that one group received treatment and then completed a posttest observation and measurement step. The other group, represented by the sequence R O, completed only the posttest measurement step. The control group in this example is a *no treatment control* rather than an alternate treatment control.

However, researchers often want to compare two different treatments or experimental manipulations rather than treatment and no treatment conditions. The notation for a posttest-only design in which the researcher compares two treatments is slightly different, as shown below.

Example 2

Posttest-Only Randomized Treatment Groups

| R | X_1 | O |
| R | X_2 | O |

Researchers could vary this basic design in several ways. For example, they might want to compare two alternate treatments as well as a no treatment control group, as in Example 3, or they might compare three different treatments, as in Example 4.

Example 3

Posttest-Only Randomized Treatment and Control Groups

R	X_1	O
R	X_2	O
R		O

Example 4

Posttest-Only Randomized Treatment Groups (with three treatments)

R	X_1	O
R	X_2	O
R	X_3	O

Another option researchers might consider is to have a second posttest observation and measurement step (e.g., an R X O O sequence). A second posttest would provide information about the long-term effects of treatment. Audiologists and speech-language pathologists almost always obtain measures of their clients' performance before treatment and again after treatment to document progress, so you might wonder why researchers would design a study in which they test their participants only once at the end of the study. One reason to use a posttest-only design is when the researchers have reason to think giving a pretest could falsify their findings. For example, participants could learn something from the pretest that enables them to perform better on the posttest. Patten (2007) used the example of students taking a pretest over course content. These students might learn something about the topics covered in the course and focus more study time on those topics. Another possible reason to use a posttest-only design is when giving a pretest would not be feasible. An example of this might be research conducted with some type of emergency medical procedure. Perhaps medical researchers have reason to believe a certain drug could improve recovery of persons with traumatic injuries, if the patients receive the drug as soon as they enter the hospital. They design a study in which patients receive either standard emergency room care or the drug plus the standard care. However, the researchers decided they could not take time to pretest their patients before initiating treatment. Therefore, they planned to use a posttest-only randomized control group design.

Pretest-Posttest Randomized Control Group Design

When considering true experimental designs, perhaps the most frequently used type is a *pretest-posttest randomized control group design* (Patten, 2007). In a pretest-posttest design, researchers observe and measure their participants' behavior twice—at the beginning of the study before participants receive treatment and again at the end of the study after participants complete the treatment step. Thus, the sequence of steps

for this design is random assignment of participants to different groups, pretest observation and measurement of both groups, implementation of treatment for one of the groups, and posttest observation and measurement of both groups. Example 5 illustrates the notation for this type of design.

Example 5

Pretest-Posttest Randomized Control Group

R	O	X	O
R	O		O

The various options that we discussed for the posttest-only design also apply to a pretest-posttest design. For example, researchers could investigate changes associated with two different treatments rather than comparing a treatment group and a no treatment control group (e.g., two treatment sequences such as $R \ O \ X_1 \ O$ and $R \ O \ X_2 O$). They also could compare two alternate treatments as well as a no treatment control group; or they might compare three different treatments, as in Examples 6 and 7 below.

Example 6

Pretest-Posttest Randomized Treatment and Control Groups

R	O	X_1	O
R	O	X_2	O
R	O		O

Example 7

Pretest-Posttest Randomized Treatment Group (with three treatments)

R	O	X_1	O
R	O	X_2	O
R	O	X_3	O

Pretest-posttest designs are sometimes called *mixed model* designs. The pretest-posttest comparison involves repeated measures of the same participants, sometimes described as a *within-subjects* factor. The treatment-no treatment comparison involves measures from different participants, or a *between-subjects* factor. Mixed designs combine within-subjects and between-subjects factors and are well suited to investigations of treatment effects.

One of the major advantages of a pretest-posttest design is that the pretest provides evidence that the two groups were not significantly different before you initiated treatment. Thus, any group differences observed at the end of the study can be attributed to the treatment. Although random assignment of participants to groups is a way to avoid systematic variation between treatment and control groups, it is not a way to assure that the two groups are equivalent. By chance, researchers could create two groups that varied on a relevant skill at the beginning of the study. If the control group started the study with greater skill on the outcome measure, the preexisting difference could mask a treatment effect. On the other hand, if the treatment group started the study with greater skill on the outcome measure, the preexisting difference could create a false treatment effect. Thus, when choosing a posttest-only or a pretest-posttest design, researchers need to weight the relative merits of identifying any preexisting differences against the possibility that learning from the pretest could contaminate their findings.

Solomon Randomized Four-Group Design

One of the most sophisticated true experimental designs is a *Solomon randomized four-group design* (Patten, 2007). This design combines features of a posttest-only design and a pretest-posttest design. By using features of both designs, researchers have a way

to check for pretest learning effects as well as to determine if treatment and control groups were different before the researchers initiated treatment. Example 8 illustrates the structure of Solomon four-group design.

Example 8

Solomon Randomized Four-Group

R	O	X	O
R	O		O
R		X	O
R			O

A Solomon four-group design has two treatment groups represented by the R O X O and R X O sequences, and two control groups represented by the R O O and R O sequences. In interpreting this design, researchers would identify treatment effects if the participants in the two treatment groups improved more from pretest to posttest than participants in the control groups. On the other hand, if both pretest groups, represented by R O X O and R O O, improved more than the posttest-only groups, that would mean participants were learning something from the pretest that enabled them to perform better on the posttest. A Solomon four-group design is a robust design for investigating treatment effects because a researcher has ways to evaluate both pretest learning and pretreatment group differences. The major disadvantage of this design is that researchers must recruit a much larger number of participants than in a posttest-only design or a pretest-posttest design.

Switching Replications Design

Trochim and Donnelly (2007) described one additional design that is of interest for conducting intervention research. In a *switching replications design*, the participants are randomly assigned to treatment and control groups to start the study. After the first posttest, the participants switch roles; the treatment group becomes the control group and the control group becomes the treatment group for the second phase of the study. Trochim and Donnelly noted that this design is an important one to consider when conducting treatment research because " . . . it addresses one of the major problems in experimental designs: the need to deny the program to some participants through random assignment" (pp. 204–205). Trochom and Donnelly (p. 205) diagrammed this design as follows:

Example 9

Switching Replications Design

R	O	X	O		O
R	O		O	X	O

Factorial Designs

The final type of true experimental design that we will cover is a *factorial design*. In a factorial design, the researchers plan to manipulate two or more independent variables simultaneously (e.g., Rosenthal & Rosnow, 2008; Trochim & Donnelly, 2007). When describing factorial designs, we could say that each of the independent variables is a factor, and each factor has two or more levels. By using a factorial design, researchers can determine how more than one independent variable impacts a dependent variable, plus they can determine how the two independent variables work together or influence one another.

Factorial designs actually are like a family of research designs with many possible variations. The following examples will illustrate some of the options. The simplest factorial design is one with two independent variables and two levels for each of these variables. This simple design is often referred to as a 2 by 2 factorial design. An example of this design would be a treatment study in which speech-language pathologists (SLPs) investigate two different intervention approaches as well as two different intervention schedules. Let's assume that the SLPs compare a traditional intervention with a new intervention they created. In addition, the SLPs want to determine if different intervention schedules would affect how much the participants improve. They plan to compare two different treatment schedules. In one schedule participants would receive intervention twice a week in 1-hour sessions. In the other schedule, participants would receive intervention four times a week in ½-hour sessions. Thus, all the participants would receive the same total amount of treatment. In this example the two independent variables are intervention approach and schedule; the two levels of the intervention variable are the traditional and new approaches; and the two levels of the schedule variables are four ½-hour long sessions and two 1-hour long sessions.

To illustrate this factorial design, we are going to use a table rather than our notation system. The 2 by 2 intervention we described above is shown in Table 6–1. In the example, the SLPs recruited 40 individuals with speech and language disorders as participants and randomly assigned them to four different treatment options. One group received traditional intervention four times per week in ½-hour sessions; a second group received traditional intervention two times per week in 1-hour sessions; a third group received the new intervention four times per week in ½-hour sessions; and the fourth group received the new intervention two times per week in 1-hour sessions.

In this 2 by 2 factorial design, the researchers obtain information about the effects of two different independent vari-

Table 6–1. An illustration of a 2 by 2 factorial design

Schedule	Type of Intervention	
	Traditional Approach	**New Approach**
Four ½-hour sessions	Ten randomly assigned participants receive the traditional approach in four ½-hour sessions.	Ten randomly assigned participants receive the new approach in four ½-hour sessions.
Two 1-hour sessions	Ten randomly assigned participants receive the traditional approach in two 1-hour sessions.	Ten randomly assigned participants receive the new approach in two 1-hour sessions.

ables. The effects associated with each of the independent variables are called *main effects*. In our example, if the participants who received the new intervention improved more than those who received traditional intervention, no matter how intervention was scheduled, you could describe the finding as a main effect of intervention. If the participants who received intervention in four ½-hour sessions per week improved more than those who received intervention in two 1-hour sessions per week, no matter what intervention approach they received, you could describe the finding as a main effect of schedule.

An important advantage of factorial designs is that researchers can investigate not only the effect of each independent variable, but also how independent variables work together or influence one another. The effects associated with the way the independent variables work together are called *interaction effects*. Interaction effects occur in a factorial research design when the outcomes associated with one independent variable are different depending on the level of the other independent variable. An example of an interaction in our hypothetical study would be if the four ½-hour ses-

sions produced more improvement than the two 1-hour sessions, but only for the participants who received the new intervention approach. Let's make this example more concrete by using some numerical values in our illustration. For instance, both the group that received traditional intervention in ½-hour sessions and the group that received traditional intervention in 1-hour sessions improved by an average of 10 points at the end of the study. The group that received the new intervention in 1-hour sessions also improved by an average of 10 points at the end of the study; however, the group that received the new intervention in ½-hour sessions improved by 20 points. The presence of an interaction influences how you interpret your findings. In the above example, the SLPs would not be able to say that their new approach was significantly better overall; rather, their new approach was significantly better when delivered in four ½-hour sessions per week.

Like other true experimental designs, researchers have many options when creating a factorial design. For example, they could devise an independent variable with three or more levels, such as in a 2 by 3 factorial design. This type of design is illustrated in Table 6–2. In this example, the independent variables are speech recognition task and hearing aid orientation program. A group of audiologists wanted to investigate how well listeners with new hearing aid prescriptions performed on different speech recognition tasks. They also wanted to determine if an extended orientation program would improve the listeners' performance on any or all of the tasks. The speech recognition task variable had three levels, and the orientation program had two levels. With this design the researchers will be able to investigate two main effects, speech recognition task and orientation program, as well as the interaction between speech recognition task and orientation program.

Our next example is a factorial design with three independent variables. To illustrate this design we will return to our first example, investigating the effects of intervention approach and schedule. However, the SLPs who conducted the study decided to add a third variable, provision of a home program. This variable also has two levels: no home program and home program. The design shown in Table 6–3 is a 2 by 2 by 2 factorial design.

Although a factorial design provides a way to investigate several independent variables at the same time, one of the disadvantages of these designs is the need to recruit a relatively large number of participants. In our 2 by 2 by 2 factorial design, the researchers would need to recruit 80 participants to randomly assign 10 individuals to each of the possible treatment, schedule, and home program combinations. This is twice the number of participants in the basic 2 by 2 factorial design in our first example (see Table 6–1). In addition, the interaction effects become quite complex each time you add another independent variable. In the 2 by 2 by 2 design, the researchers created eight different combinations of treatment approach, schedule, and home program. A three-way interaction would arise if just one of these combinations stood out as the most effective. For our basic 2 by 2 example, we described an interaction effect in which the group that received the new intervention in ½-hour sessions improved by 20 points, as compared to a 10-point improvement for all of the other treatment and schedule combinations. To illustrate a possible three-way interaction,

Table 6–2. An illustration of a 2 by 3 factorial design

Speech Recognition Task	Type of Orientation Program	
	Regular Orientation	*Extended Orientation*
Task One	Ten randomly assigned participants complete task one after a regular orientation.	Ten randomly assigned participants complete task one after an extended orientation.
Task Two	Ten randomly assigned participants complete task two after a regular orientation.	Ten randomly assigned participants complete task two after an extended orientation.
Task Three	Ten randomly assigned participants complete task three after a regular orientation.	Ten randomly assigned participants complete task three after an extended orientation.

Table 6–3. An illustration of a 2 by 2 by 2 factorial design

	Provision of Home Program			
	No Home Program		Home Program	
	Type of Intervention		Type of Intervention	
Schedule	Traditional Approach	New Approach	Traditional Approach	New Approach
Four ½-hour sessions	Ten randomly assigned participants receive the traditional approach in four ½-hour sessions with no home program.	Ten randomly assigned participants receive the new approach in four ½-hour sessions with no home program.	Ten randomly assigned participants receive the traditional approach in four ½-hour sessions with a home program.	Ten randomly assigned participants receive the new approach in four ½-hour sessions with a home program.
Two 1-hour sessions	Ten randomly assigned participants receive the traditional approach in two 1-hour sessions with no home program.	Ten randomly assigned participants receive the new approach in two 1-hour sessions with no home program.	Ten randomly assigned participants receive the traditional approach in two 1-hour sessions with a home program.	Ten randomly assigned participants receive the new approach in two 1-hour sessions with a home program.

let's consider those participants who received the new treatment approach scheduled in ½-hour sessions four times per week. The 2 by 2 by 2 design includes two groups with this combination. One group received a home program and the other did not. Perhaps, the group that received the combination of new treatment approach scheduled in ½-hour sessions four times per week plus a home program performed the best at the end of the study, gaining an average of 30 points on the posttest. In comparison, the group that received the combination of new treatment approach scheduled in ½-hour sessions four times per week with no home program gained 20 points. This would be an example of a three-way interaction, because both schedule and the provision of a home program interacted with treatment approach.

Deciding how many independent variables to investigate is one of the major decisions researchers make when planning a study with a factorial design. However, they need to consider other features too, such as whether to use a posttest-only design or a pretest-posttest design. They also might decide to conduct a long-term follow-up and include a second posttest observation in their research plan. Another possibility is to use a factorial design that combines experimental and nonexperimental variables. That is, researchers might decide to investigate one or more variables that they manipulate during the study and other variables that are preexisting conditions. One example of this would be to investigate an experimental variable such as intervention approach, and a nonexperimental variable such as severity of disorder. This example is illustrated in Table 6–4 and is a modification of the example presented in Table 6–1. However, in Table 6–4, the researchers plan to investigate the effectiveness of the traditional and new intervention approaches with participants who have mild-to-moderate or severe speech and language disorders. The researchers can still assign participants to the intervention approaches on a random basis, but the severity levels involve preexisting conditions that cannot be assigned at random.

Each design we covered in this section is a true experimental design. The designs are true experiments as long as the researchers manipulate at least one of the independent variables, exercising experimental control over this variable, and randomly assign participants to the different levels of this variable. These two criteria, random assignment

Table 6–4. An illustration of a 2 by 2 factorial design with experimental and nonexperiment independent variables

Level of Severity	Type of Intervention	
	Traditional Approach	*New Approach*
Mild-to-Moderate Disorders	Ten participants with mild-to-moderate disorders randomly assigned to receive the traditional approach	Ten participants with mild-to-moderate disorders randomly assigned to receive the new approach
Severe Disorders	Ten participants with severe disorders randomly assigned to receive the traditional approach	Ten participants with severe disorders randomly assigned to receive the new approach

to groups and experimental manipulation of an independent variable, are essential for investigating cause and effect relationships. If researchers want to demonstrate that a new intervention approach led to significant improvement for their participants, they need to design a study in which they randomly assign participants to this new intervention and to at least one other group, such as a no treatment control group or an alternate treatment group. Their experimental manipulation will be the type of treatment the participants receive. When researchers combine experimental and nonexperimental variables in a factorial study, they will be able to a demonstrate cause and effect relationship only for the experimental variable. The results from the nonexperimental comparison do not support conclusions about cause and effect, although information about the nonexperimental variable and how it interacts with the experimental manipulation could be important.

Research using true experimental designs is crucially important to professionals in audiology and speech-language pathology who provide treatment for individuals with communication disorders. Any clinical field that provides treatment services needs evidence to demonstrate the effectiveness of those services, and the strongest evidence for cause and effect relationships comes from true experimental research. The research base for audiology and speech-language pathology certainly includes a number of studies with both experimental manipulation of treatment variables and random assignment of participants to two or more groups. A few recent examples include studies addressing different treatment programs for persons with aphasia (Doesborgh et al., 2003; Elman & Bernstein-Ellis, 1999), an aural rehabilitation program for persons recently fitted with a hearing aid (Chisolm,

Abrams, & McArdle, 2004), treatment of children's phonological disorders (Almost & Rosenbaum, 1998), a phonemic awareness training program for children with speech disorders (Hesketh, Dima, & Nelson, 2007), use of sound field amplification in classrooms (Mendel, Roberts, & Walton, 2003), treatment approaches for children who stutter (Hancock et al., 1998; Harris, Onslow, Packman, Harrison, & Menzies, 2002), and treatment focusing on vocabulary growth of young children (Kouri, 2005).

Importance of Experimental Control

Given the challenges of implementing a true experimental design, potential researchers might wonder about its importance. One reason researchers try to implement a true experimental design is to increase the validity of their conclusions regarding cause and effect relationships. If a study lacks a control group, or the participants were not randomly assigned, the case for a cause and effect relationship between the independent variable and observed changes in the dependent variable is weak. The reason is that a number of alternative explanations, called *threats to internal validity*, could be the source of the changes in the dependent measure. Internal validity refers to the extent to which researchers' conclusions about cause and effect relationships are accurate (Patten, 2007; Trochim & Donnelly, 2007). For example, if some researchers observed that their participants scored significantly higher on a posttest outcome measure compared to the pretest scores, the researcher would like to conclude that this improvement occurred because of the treatment provided during their experiment. However, if the study lacked a control group, other possible causes of the improvement might exist that were unknown to the researchers. To illustrate these possible alternative explanations, several of the most common threats to internal validity are described in the following sections.

History

The threat of *history* means that some outside influence occurred during the course of your study, and this outside influence could account for the changes in outcome you observed at the end of your study. This threat might occur if researchers tried to conduct an intervention or training study using a single group of participants. For instance, the researchers might conduct their study with a group of students randomly selected from the same classroom. During the course of their study, the classroom teacher implemented some changes in her teaching methods and these changes addressed the same skills as the experimental training program the researchers were investigating. Because of this historical threat, the researchers would not know if their participants' improvements were due to the experimental manipulation or the classroom teacher's new methods. This alternate explanation for why the participants improved weakens any claims the researchers might make about the benefits of their experimental training program.

Maturation

The threat of *maturation* refers to increases in performance that are due to the participants' growth and development over time. This threat is particularly important when conducting research with children. However, audiologists and speech-language pathol-

ogists might consider the possibility of recovery over time as a special form of the maturation threat. Both growth and development and recovery mean that participants make improvement from pretest to posttest even without treatment. As with most threats to internal validity, the primary way to control for the maturation threat is to include a control group as well as an experimental treatment group in your design. If the treatment group improves more than the control group from pretest to posttest, researchers have evidence that growth and maturation alone cannot account for their results.

Statistical Regression

In some experimental research, researchers recruit and select participants because they performed very poorly on some prestudy selection measure. This selection measure might also serve as the pretest measure for those participants who complete the study. A phenomenon called *statistical regression* occurs when persons who scored very high or very low on a test are retested (Patton, 2007). Those who received extreme scores when first tested tend to score closer to the mean when retested. Any individual who takes a test repeatedly will exhibit some variability in her scores. If the person scored close to the mean to begin, then the scores can vary up or down. However, Trochim and Donnelly (2007) noted that persons who score either extremely high or extremely low have a strong probability of scoring closer to the mean because that is the only direction their scores can move. If you already had an extremely low score on a test, the possibility of achieving an even lower score on retest is remote, but the possibility of achieving a higher score is relatively good. Those who are extremely low will tend to score higher just based on statistical averages, and those who score extremely high would tend to score lower. The threat of statistical regression is important for treatment studies, because one of the selection criteria is that participants exhibit some deficiency on the skill that is the focus of the study. On average, the participants would tend to score higher on a posttest due to the phenomenon of statistical regression toward the mean, even if they received no benefit from the experimental treatment. This is why including a control group or an alternate treatment group in intervention research is extremely important.

Instrumentation

An *instrumentation* threat is possible in any pretest-posttest design. This threat encompasses both physical equipment used to elicit, record, and analyze responses as well as human "instruments" who observe and record behaviors. An instrumentation threat is operating in a study when the instrument changes in some way between the pretest and posttest. Thus, any differences in the participants' scores occur because of the instrumentation change rather than a treatment effect. Changes in how human observers score or measure behaviors could occur because of learning from pretest to posttest, or because of fatigue or boredom with the task. If observers learn over the course of the study and become more accurate in identifying relevant behaviors, participants' scores might be higher at the end of the study due to observer changes rather than due to a real treatment effect. If observers become fatigued or bored, they could become less accurate or vigilant from pretest to posttest. Failure to properly maintain calibration of a piece of equipment and an undiscovered equipment defect that

occurred between the pretest and posttest also are examples of the instrumentation threat. The inadequate calibration or equipment defect could either create a false treatment effect or mask a treatment effect that actually existed. The best way to control for an instrumentation threat is to choose a research design with a control or alternate treatment group, because the instrumentation problem will affect both the treatment and control groups. Additionally, researchers generally are careful about the calibration and maintenance of any physical instruments used in their studies.

Selection

A selection threat occurs when two or more groups differ in a systematic way, rather than in a random way, prior to a study (Patton, 2007). Groups might differ in a systematic way if the researchers select their treatment and control groups in a nonrandom way. For example, researchers might want to conduct a study that involves a classroom intervention or even a community intervention (Trochim & Donnelly, 2007). Randomly assigning children to classrooms or individuals to communities is not practical. In these cases, researchers often work with the existing or "intact groups" when conducting a study (Patten, 2007). One of the existing groups receives the experimental treatment and the other serves as a control. Studies of this type are not true experiments and the findings might be shaped by group differences unrelated to the study. Any conclusions about cause and effect relationships are weakened because of possible alternate explanations for the findings. For example, a selection threat might co-occur with maturation differences (Trochim & Donnelly, 2007). One of the groups might have a different learning or growth rate prior to the study. Over the course of the study this group will continue to improve at a faster rate than the other group. This difference in rate of improvement would be an alternate explanation for group differences observed at the end of the study. A selection threat might also co-occur with differences in group history. If researchers conduct a study with intact classrooms, differences in how the teachers teach their classes over the course of the study could be an alternate explanation. Thus, whenever it is feasible, researchers employ a true experimental design and randomly assign their participants to the treatment and control groups.

Mortality

Some threats to the internal validity of experimental research cannot be eliminated through random assignment of participants to groups. A *mortality* threat occurs when some participants drop out before the end of a study. This could occur whether the researchers used random assignment to form groups or worked with preexisting groups. If participants dropped out of the study on a random basis, mortality would be less of a threat. However, sometimes participants have a reason for dropping out of a study and this reason could distort the findings in some way. For example, participants who receive low scores on the pretest might withdraw from the study because they perceive themselves as doing poorly. In a treatment study, participants who experience less benefit from the treatment might be more likely to withdraw than those who perceive themselves as improving. If partic-

ipants drop out in a systematic way, such as those who score low on the pretest or those who are making less improvement, then the results of the study might misrepresent the true effectiveness of the treatment. If only the high scorers or those who make the most progress remain in the study for the posttest, the treatment would seem more successful than it actually is. Trochim and Donnelly (2007) suggested one way to investigate the impact of participant mortality is to compare the pretest scores of those who withdraw from the study and those who remain. If these scores are similar, then pretest differences probably are not a factor. However, comparing pretest scores would not be a way to control for different treatment experiences.

Quasi-Experimental Approaches

For some kinds of research, randomly assigning participants to treatment and control groups would be impractical. In the social sciences, researchers sometimes investigate the effectiveness of an intervention program provided to an entire community or organization (Trochim & Donnelly, 2007). In the field of education, researchers often implement and study innovative teaching and learning practices at the classroom level.[2] In these instances, randomly assigning participants to groups is not feasible. Researchers interested in community-, organizational-, or classroom-based interventions still have ways to conduct their studies, but they must do so with preexisting groups of participants. If researchers design a study in which they create different conditions or

---

[2]In some educational research, many classrooms participate in the research and the investigators randomly assign several classrooms to the experimental and control conditions. These types of studies are true experimental research. In a sense, the classrooms are a variable in the study and the students are described as being "nested" within the classrooms (Kennedy, 1978). These sophisticated designs are beyond the scope of this chapter.

experiences for the participants by manipulating some factor, but use existing groups rather than randomly formed groups, the design is a *quasi-experimental design*. Quasi-experimental designs have one of the features of a true experiment, researcher manipulation of a variable, but lack the second feature of random assignment of participants to different experimental groups (Patten, 2007; Trochim & Donnelly, 2007). Quasi-experimental designs are valuable for investigating cause and effect relationships but are more susceptible to threats to internal validity, and particularly to the selection threat. This means that conclusions regarding cause and effect relationships drawn from quasi-experimental research are weaker than those drawn from true experimental research. In the sections that follow, we discuss some of the options researchers use when a true experimental design is impractical.

Nonequivalent Control Group Designs

When the plan of a study involves identifying two preexisting or intact groups, assigning one of the groups to an experimental treatment condition and assigning the other to a control or alternate treatment condition, the design is a *nonequivalent control group design*. When using this design, researchers sometimes randomly assign one of the groups to the experimental condition and the other to the control condition. However, randomly assigning intact groups does not eliminate the problems associated with using intact groups and is not the same as randomly assigning individual participants to groups, although it might reduce researcher bias in deciding who receives the experimental treatment. A nonequivalent control group design is usually a pretest-posttest design rather than a posttest-only design. The reason for this is that the researchers have

a greater need to determine if the groups were similar on the relevant variables before treatment. Unlike groups formed at random, intact groups might be systematically different before the study due to different prior experiences, different learning and maturation rates, and so forth. Thus, researchers usually administer a pretest to demonstrate that the groups were not significantly different before the study, at least on the tested variables.

The design notation for a quasi-experimental study is similar to that for a pretest-posttest randomized control study, except that use of an R to designate random assignment is inappropriate. In the design notation, the R for group assignment might be omitted (Patten, 2007), or an N might be used for nonrandom assignment of participants to groups (Trochim & Donnelly, 2007), as we do in the examples that follow. Example 10 illustrates a basic nonequivalent control group design, and Example 11 illustrates a design with both an alternate treatment group and a no treatment control group. The primary difference between these designs and their true experimental counterparts is that the researchers are working with existing groups that were formed prior to the study for other purposes.

Example 10

Pretest-Posttest Nonequivalent Control Group

N	O	X	O
N	O		O

Example 11

Pretest-Posttest Nonequivalent Treatment and Control Groups

N	O	X_1	O
N	O	X_2	O
N	O		O

A nonequivalent control group design could be combined with the switching replications design described in Trochim and Donnelly (2007). As with any intervention study, researchers are often hesitant to withhold an innovative teaching practice that has the potential to genuinely improve student learning. In the switching replications design, both groups eventually have an opportunity to experience the innovative method, and if the approach works both during the initial implementation and during the replication, the researchers have stronger evidence for a cause and effect relationship. A nonequivalent control group design with switching replications is illustrated in Example 12.

Example 12

Switching Replications Design with Nonequivalent Control Group

N	O	X	O		O
N	O		O	X	O

One additional quasi-experimental design to consider, particularly when conducting an intervention study, is a *double pretest* design (Trochim & Donnelly, 2007). In this design, the researchers select two existing groups of participants. One group of participants receives an experimental intervention, whereas the other group participates in a no-treatment control condition or receives an alternate intervention. Example 13 provides an illustration of a double pretest design with nonrandom assignment of participants to groups (Trochim & Donnelly, p. 225).

Example 13

Double Pretest-Posttest Nonequivalent Control Group

N	O	O	X	O
N	O	O		O

The primary advantage of a double pretest design is that it provides some control over the selection threat associated with different rates of maturation or learning. If the rates of learning of two groups differed, the groups might not be significantly different at the time of the first pretest but could be significantly different at the time of the posttest. If the researchers had only obtained the first pretest, they might have assumed the two groups were similar and the differences they observed after the experimental intervention were due to the intervention. Having the second pretest could provide evidence that the scores of the two groups were diverging before the experimental intervention occurred. On the other hand, if the groups were not significantly different on either the first or the second pretest, the researchers have a stronger basis for concluding that differences observed at the end of the study were due to their experimental intervention.

Repeated Measures Group Design

Another option researchers might consider is to design an experimental study with only one group of participants. In a *repeated measures design*, researchers obtain two or more measurements from the same participants. Sometimes repeated measures designs are nonexperimental in nature, and researchers obtain a series of measurements across time to observe participants' maturation or learning in an area of interest. However, repeated measures designs can be experimental designs as well. In a repeated measures experimental design, participants serve as their own controls and experience all levels of the independent variable. Thus, we will classify this design as a quasi-experimental rather than a true experimental design, because participants are not randomly assigned to treatment and control groups. The advantages of using a repeated measures design, compared to randomized pretest-posttest designs, are that researchers do not need to recruit as many participants and the experimental and control groups are well matched because participants serve as their own controls. However, a repeated measures experimental design is only feasible in situations where the order of the experimental and control conditions will not affect outcomes. Further, researchers need to be aware of challenges in analyzing the findings from repeated measures experiments, particularly when participants are observed and measured three or more times (Max & Onghena, 1999).

Previously, we noted that some experimental manipulations are actual interventions designed to increase participants' abilities and skills. Other experimental manipulations are task manipulations designed to increase participants' performance at that moment, but not necessarily to increase the performance in a permanent way. A repeated measures design could work quite well with the latter type of independent variable, but probably is not well suited to actual intervention research. For example, researchers in audiology might want to compare two different amplification approaches for persons with hearing losses. They could randomly assign participants to the two amplification conditions, but this might not be practical if the number of participants who fit the researchers' criteria for participation was small. As an alternative, the researchers could test each of the participants twice, giving each participant an opportunity to try both amplification approaches. As another example, researchers might be interested in an interaction variable that might alter children's communication in a temporary way, perhaps promoting greater fluency or more talkativeness. The researchers might design a study in which the children participated for part of the time in the experimental condition and part of the time in the control condition. Even if the children participated in the experimental condition first, the expectation is that their conversational participation or fluency would return to typical levels in the control condition. Example 14 below shows the simplest form of a repeated measures design with one group of participants who experience both the experimental (X_1) and control conditions (X_2).

Example 14

Repeated Measures Experimental Design

$$X_1 \qquad O \qquad X_2 \qquad O$$

Often researchers increase the experimental control in repeated measures studies by counterbalancing the order of experimental and control conditions. Counterbalancing works well when the independent variable has two levels. Half of the participants complete the experimental condition first, followed by the control condition, whereas the remaining half complete the control condition followed by the experimental condition. Counterbalancing provides the researchers with a way to identify any order effects in their outcomes. Example 15 is an illustration of a repeated measures design with counterbalancing and random assignment to order of experimental and control experiences. In the example below, half of the participants undergo experimental treatment first followed by an alternate treatment control condition; the other half undergo the alternate treatment first followed by the experimental treatment. The R designates random assignment to order of treatment, but not to treatment or control conditions, because all participants experience both treatment options.

Example 15

Repeated Measures Experimental Design with Counterbalancing

$$R \qquad X_1 \qquad O \qquad X_2 \qquad O$$
$$R \qquad X_2 \qquad O \qquad X_1 \qquad O$$

Repeated measures designs are also referred to as within-subject designs. This means that individual participants experience the different levels or the independent variable or treatment and control conditions (Shearer, 1997). Repeated measures designs are a viable option for investigating some questions in the field of communication sciences and disorders, as demonstrated in several recent studies (e.g., Chapman, Sindberg, Bridge, Gigstead, & Hesketh, 2006; Cherry & Rubinstein, 2006; Gordon-Salant, Fitzgibbons, & Friedman, 2007; Ilgaz & Aksu-Koc, 2005).

Thus far, both the true experimental and quasi-experimental designs covered in this section have been group designs. In group designs researchers report results for an average or typical member of a group (Silverman, 1998), as well as the spread of scores from low to high among group members. Although researchers might occasionally identify a member of a group who performed in an atypical way, usually the focus is on the collective performance of a group and not the performance of individual participants. Group designs are a dominant approach in many fields of study, including audiology and speech-language pathology. However, group designs might not be feasible for studying certain research questions. If the number of potential participants is relatively small, such as in research focusing on treatment for a disorder with low prevalence, a group design often is not the best choice. A group design also is less suitable when researchers might expect participants to respond in distinctive ways to their treatment (Silverman, 1998). When participant responses are highly individualistic, discussing findings in terms of the typical or average performance of a group is inappropriate. In the next section, we cover alternative, single subject designs, which might be more appropriate in situations where

the population of participants is small or participants' responses to the experimental manipulation are likely to be highly variable.

Single Subject Designs

In research that employs a *single subject design*, researchers report the results for each individual participant separately. The term single subject design refers to how researchers report their findings and does not mean that the study had only one participant in a literal sense (Silverman, 1998). In fact, researchers often replicate their approach with two or more participants. Single subject designs fit the category of quasi-experimental designs because such designs have one or more experimental manipulations but lack random assignment of participants to groups. Like in repeated measures designs, participants in single subject research experience both treatment and control conditions. The difference is that researchers report the combined results for all participants with repeated measures designs but report the results for individual participants with single subject designs.

Often the notation system for single subject designs employs the letters A, B, C, and so forth (e.g., Barlow & Hersen, 1984; Leary, 2001; McReynolds & Kearns, 1983; Richards, Taylor, Ramasamy, & Richards, 1999). The letter A designates a baseline or no treatment phase in a study, and the letter B designates the first treatment approach. If the study includes more than one treatment approach, the letter C designates the second treatment approach or sometimes designates a second element of treatment that combines with B (McReynolds & Kearns, 1983). To establish a functional relationship between a treatment and behavioral change, researchers measure the target behavior many times over a series of sessions. If the behavior remains relatively stable during the baseline, no treatment phase, and changes in a noticeable way during the treatment phase, the researchers have evidence for a relationship between the treatment and the change in behavior.

The simplest single subject design is an A-B sequence, or a baseline-treatment design. Although an A-B sequence is the basis for all other single subject designs, the design itself is rather weak and seldom found in reported research (Richards et al., 1999). Because the design includes only one A and one B phase, any changes that occur during the B phase could have alternative explanations such as maturation or an extraneous environmental change. However, this simple single subject design does have utility for audiologists and speech-language pathologists who need to document the effectiveness of their interventions for persons with speech, language, and hearing impairments.

A more sophisticated modification of an A-B design is an A_1-B-A_2 or *treatment withdrawal* design (Barlow & Hersen, 1984), also sometimes called a reversal design (Leary, 2001). The subscripts on A_1 and A_2 indicate whether the baseline phase was the first or second in the series. In this design, researchers collect baseline data during a no treatment phase first (A_1), implement an experimental intervention for several sessions, and then withdraw the intervention and collect data during a second no treatment phase (A_2). This design provides additional evidence for a functional (cause and effect) relationship between the experimental intervention and observed behavioral changes, if the behavior in the second baseline phase returns to levels observed during the first baseline phase. Consider the example of audiologists who want to test the effectiveness of an experimental amplification approach. They would collect baseline data by testing a participant without the

experimental amplification for perhaps a minimum of three sessions; next they would implement the amplification phase for several sessions, and then withdraw the amplification and test the participant for three additional baseline sessions. This hypothetical design is illustrated in Figure 6–1. In this figure, the vertical lines inserted between the A and B phases indicate the switch from no treatment baseline to treatment phases. In this idealized experimental illustration, the behavior remained stable during the initial three baseline sessions, the behavior immediately increased and stayed at a high level when treatment was implemented for eight sessions, and finally the behavior returned to pretreatment levels during the second set of three baseline sessions. A treatment withdrawal design is appropriate when investigating experimental interventions you expect to affect the target behavior only while the experimental intervention is occurring. With interventions that have a temporary effect, the participant's behavior should return to A_1 baseline levels once the intervention is no longer present. If the target behavior returns to levels present during the first baseline phase, you have evidence that the change in behavior resulted from the experimental intervention. If the target behavior remained at treatment levels after treatment withdrawal, the change in behavior could be attributed to some extraneous factor and the evidence for a treatment effect is weakened. For this reason, an A_1-B-A_2 design is not ideal for interventions that create lasting changes in the target behavior, because behaviors should remain at or near the levels present during the B or intervention phase.

Another modification of a simple baseline-treatment design is a *treatment replication* or A_1-B_1-A_2-B_2 design (Richards et al., 1999). In this design, illustrated in Figure 6–2, the researcher includes two A-B series

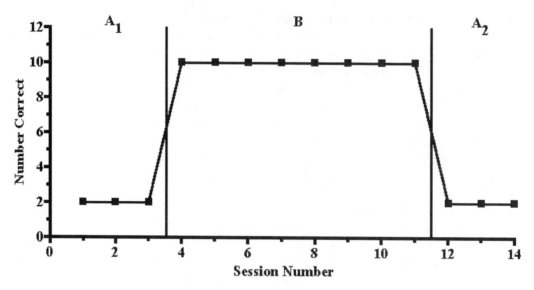

Figure 6–1. Illustration of an A_1-B-A_2 treatment withdrawal single subject design.

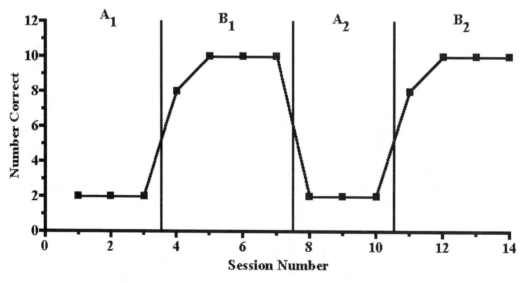

Figure 6–2. Illustration of an A_1-B_1-A_2-B_2 treatment replication single subject design in which measured behaviors returned to initial baseline levels during the second baseline phase.

to determine if effects that appear to be associated with treatment during the first phase can be repeated during a second treatment phase. After measuring behaviors dur-

ing several baseline sessions, the investigator introduces an intervention and measures behaviors during several intervention sessions. Then, the investigator repeats the series by withdrawing intervention during a second baseline phase and reintroducing intervention during a second treatment series. If the behaviors return to baseline levels when intervention is withdrawn and change again when the intervention is reintroduced, the investigator has strong evidence that the intervention was the cause of the behavior change. If the behaviors do not return to baseline levels when intervention is withdrawn but change even more in a second intervention phase, such as illustrated in Figure 6–3, the evidence for a cause and effect relationship between intervention and the behavior change is still relatively strong. On the other hand, if behaviors measured in the second baseline phase do not return to initial baseline levels, or the participant does not show any improvement in the second intervention, the evidence for a functional, cause and effect relationship is relatively weak.

Another variation on the treatment withdrawal design is a *multiple treatment*

design. This design begins with an A_1-B_1-A_2 series, but instead of following this with a second phase of the B intervention (B_2), the researchers implement a new intervention (e.g., C) (Leary, 2001; Richards et al., 1999). This notation for a multiple treatment design would be A_1-B-A_2-C, and often researchers follow C with a third baseline phase, A_1-B-A_2-C-A_3. Although this design allows the researchers to investigate the effects of a second treatment, the design does not provide evidence for the effectiveness of the C treatment by itself, only its effectiveness following prior administration of the B treatment. This is a serial order confound because the C treatment followed the B. Sometimes researchers employ this design with two or more participants and counterbalance the order. That is, one participant experiences the sequence A_1-B-A_2-C-A_3, whereas the other experiences the sequence A_1-C-A_2-B-A_3.

The basic single subject baseline-treatment design can be extended in many

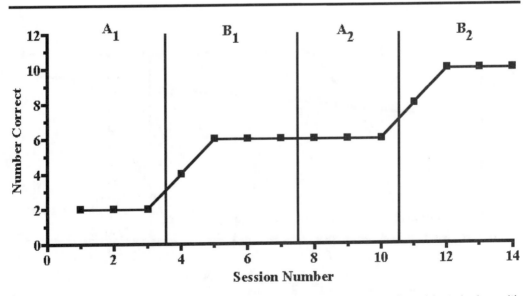

Figure 6–3. Illustration of an A_1-B_1-A_2-B_2 treatment replication single subject design with incremental treatment effects in both B_1 and B_2 treatment phases.

ways and we have covered only a few of those options (Barlow & Hersen, 1984; Kratochwill, 1992; Richards et al., 1999). For example, researchers sometimes extend the treatment replication design for several A-B series or rapidly alternate treatment and baseline every other session. Sometimes two treatment components are combined at the same time and designated as a BC phase.

Another alternative to strengthen the experimental control in a single subject design is to use a *multiple baseline* design. Some of the common variations are multiple baseline across participants, behaviors, and settings (Barlow & Hersen, 1984; McReynolds & Thompson, 1986; Richards et al., 1999). In a *multiple baseline across behaviors* design, researchers select two or more behaviors to observe and measure during the study. They determine baseline levels for both behaviors during the initial baseline phase and then initiate treatment for one of the behaviors. They continue to observe and measure the second behavior but do

not immediately initiate treatment on that behavior. Sometimes the researchers continue to measure this behavior only, but often they begin treatment on this second behavior during a second treatment phase.

In the example illustrated in Figure 6-4, the researchers created two equivalent word lists. These could be lists of new vocabulary items, lists of words with speech sounds to discriminate, or other ideas you might generate. The researchers obtained baseline levels for both lists during the A_1 phase and then initiated treatment with the first word list. At the same time, they continued to observe the participant's performance with the second word list. You might think of this as an extended baseline phase for list 2. In this particular example, the improvements that occurred for list 1 words in the first treatment phase (B_1) were maintained during the second baseline or treatment withdrawal phase (A_2). Although maintenance of treatment gains during the treatment withdrawal phase weakens the evidence

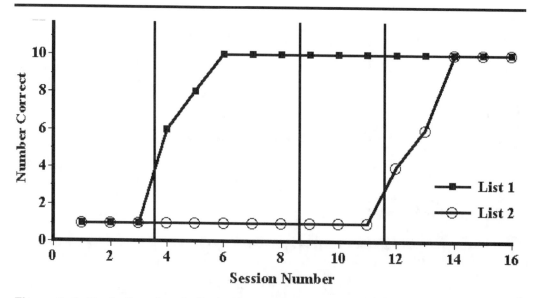

Figure 6–4. Illustration of an A_1-B_1-A_2-B_2 multiple baseline across behaviors single subject design.

for a cause and effect relationship between the treatment and behavior change, this is often the kind of pattern audiologists and speech-language pathologists want to see. That is, clinicians try to identify treatment approaches that will produce lasting improvements in their clients. Fortunately, a multiple baseline across behaviors design provides an additional opportunity for researchers to demonstrate a functional relationship between the treatment and behavior changes. For the example in Figure 6–4, the number correct for the untreated words in list 2 remained at baseline levels during the first treatment phase (B_1) and second baseline phase (A_2). For the final treatment phase (B_2), the researchers started treatment on the words in list 2, and this is the point in the study when the participant's performance with these words improved. This multiple baseline design has several sources of experimental control to strengthen the evidence for a cause and effect relationship: (a) stable baselines for both word lists during the A_1 phase; (b) improved performance on the treated words in list 1 during the B_1 phase; (c) stable baseline levels for the untreated words in list 2 through phases A_1-B_1-A_2 phases; and (d) improved performance on the words in list 2 with the initiation of treatment on those words in the B_2 phase. Because of these sources of experimental control, a multiple baseline across behaviors design is a good choice when investigating treatment approaches for speech, language, and hearing disorders.

When planning to use a multiple baseline across behaviors design, researchers need to give careful consideration to the choice of a second behavior to baseline and eventually treat. The second behavior should be generally equivalent to the first in difficulty and/or developmental level. For example, if researchers were constructing two word lists, it would be inappropriate to construct a treatment list with common, high frequency words and to construct a probe list with less common, low frequency words. Researchers also need to avoid behaviors that might change through treatment of the first behavior. One area where this is an issue is in studies that address production and perception of speech sounds. If researchers selected a second speech sound to observe and measure in the A_1-B_1-A_2 phases of treatment, they need to avoid sounds that might improve because they share phonetic features with the trained phoneme. For example, if the first trained sound was /k/, /g/ would be a poor choice as a control phoneme. Because the /k/ and /g/ share phonetic features (velar, stop), training one of these sounds could lead to improvement in the other through feature generalization (Bernthal & Bankson, 2003).

A final option covered here is a *multiple baseline across participants* (subjects) design (Barlow & Hersen, 1984; Kearns, 1986; Richards et al., 1999). In this kind of study, researchers duplicate their intervention with one or more additional participants. A multiple baseline across participants design is often combined with an A_1-B_1-A_2-B_2 treatment replication design, as shown in Figure 6–5. Each participant could start the study at the same time and begin the treatment phase at the same time, but this is not the best arrangement. If the participants start treatment at the same time, any observed improvement in the participants' behavior could be due to an extraneous source, rather than the experimental intervention. Therefore, researchers often stagger the onset of the intervention phase across participants. In the example in Figure 6–5, the first participant completed three baseline sessions and then entered the intervention phase, but the second participant completed two additional baseline sessions before beginning intervention. If the intervention

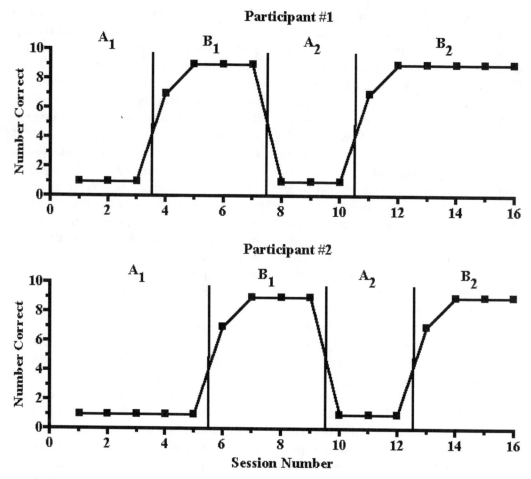

Figure 6–5. Illustration of an A_1-B_1-A_2-B_2 multiple baseline across participants single subject design.

is the cause of the observed change in the target skill, then the first participant should begin improving in sessions four and five, but the second participant should continue exhibiting baseline levels and not start improving until sessions six and seven. This is in fact the pattern illustrated in the graphs in Figure 6-5.

Single subject research designs are well suited to studying an individual's response to intervention (Leary, 2001). If individual participants respond in unique ways to the intervention, the research is still valuable because findings are not aggregated across participants. In group research, individual variability in response to intervention tends to be obscured in the averaged data.

These designs allow researchers to compare behaviors observed during baseline phases with those observed during intervention to determine if there is a functional, cause and effect relationship between an intervention and observed changes in behavior (McReynolds & Thompson, 1986). Because single subject designs provide a researcher with ways to establish experimental control, they provide stronger evidence than nonexperimental case studies. Single subject designs have a long history of use in the field of communication sciences and disorders in research with both children (e.g., Goldstein, English, Shafer, & Kaczmarek, 1997; Kashinath, Woods, & Goldstein, 2006; Scherer, 1999; Weismer, Murray-Branch, & Miller, 1993; Winslow & Guitar, 1994) and adults with communication disorders (e.g., Ballard & Thompson, 1999; Drew & Thompson, 1999; Palmer, Adams, Bourgeois, Durrant, & Rossi, 1999).

Experimental Designs and Levels of Evidence

Previously we learned that the term *evidence-based practice* (EBP) refers to an approach in which clinicians use the best available research to guide their decisions about how to evaluate and treat persons with communication disorders. Some of the steps in EBP include identifying a clinical questions, searching the professional literature, and reading and evaluating research reports.In Chapter 3 and Chapter 4, we covered developing a clinical question and conducting a literature search as the initial steps in completing evidence-based practice research. The next step after completing the literature search is to select the most relevant articles to read and evaluate. An important consideration in evaluating research is to determine the *level of evidence* a study provides, and knowledge about research design is a key factor in making this judgment. As noted previously in this chapter, the strongest designs for establishing cause and effect relationships are true experimental designs—those with random assignment of participants to at least two groups, a treatment and a control group. True experimental designs, sometimes called randomized clinical trials, provide the strongest kind of evidence for intervention effectiveness and include studies that compare treatment and no treatment conditions, as well as those that

compare two or more different treatment approaches. Other experimental designs provide useful information, but the strength of evidence for a cause and effect relationship is weaker.

In addition to level of evidence, audiologists and speech-language pathologists consider the depth of evidence that supports the effectiveness of a particular intervention approach. For example, a well-designed, randomized clinical trial is considered a strong type of evidence, and several well-designed, randomized clinical trials that yielded similar results would be even stronger. If the studies yielded conflicting results, then the evidence in support of a particular intervention approach is undermined.

Sometimes your literature search might yield a systematic review or meta-analysis. From your reading, you might be familiar with a narrative review of literature in the introduction section of research reports (Cook, Mulrow, & Haynes, 1997). A *systematic review* is a special kind of review of existing research that employs a rigorous method of evaluation. The authors of a systematic review use a specific procedure to search the research literature, select the studies to include in their review, and critically evaluate the studies they find. In addition, authors of systematic reviews usually have identified a particular clinical question to answer when they begin their literature search (Cook et al., 1997). A *meta-analysis* adds an additional component, a statistical analysis of the aggregated findings from several studies, and provides an estimate of the overall effectiveness of an intervention (Schlosser, 2006; Trochim & Donnelly, 2007). This combined estimate of effect should be less affected by random or systematic sources of bias in the individual studies and thus should be more stable.

Many organizations have published levels of evidence models to guide professionals in their evaluation of the strength of evidence obtained from different studies (e.g., American Speech-Language-Hearing Association, 2004; Centre for Evidence-Based Medicine, n.d.; Health Science Information Service, 2007). The various models have more similarities than differences. For example, nearly all models place randomized clinical trials and meta-analyses at the highest level. A randomized clinical trial represents the highest level for individual studies, and several studies combined in a meta-analysis demonstrate the depth of evidence for a particular intervention. Similarly, nearly all models place expert opinion at the lowest level. However, one might consider the convergent opinions of several experts (a panel of experts) to be stronger than the opinion of a single expert. Thus, judging the evidence in support of a particular intervention means considering the strength of the individual studies as well as the number of studies. At any level of evidence, having multiple sources that report similar findings is stronger than having a single source at that level. However, a single well-designed randomized clinical trial would generally outweigh the opinion of several experts. Figure 6–6 illustrated the concepts of strength of evidence and depth of evidence for intervention research.[3]

Finally, let's consider how the various nonexperimental and experimental research designs go with the common levels of evidence cited in the literature (American Speech-Language-Hearing Association, 2004; Centre for Evidence-Based Medicine, n.d.; Health Science Information Service, 2007). As noted previously, randomized clinical trials are at the highest level of evidence. Examples of designs that could be employed in such trials include pretest-posttest randomized treatment and control group designs, the Solomon four-group design, random-

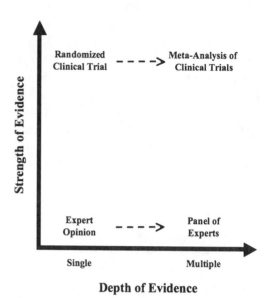

Figure 6–6. Illustration of contributions of strength and depth of research findings to decisions about levels of evidence.

ized switching replications designs, and randomized factorial designs. At the next lower level are various quasi-experimental designs with nonrandomized treatment and control groups such as a pretest-posttest nonequivalent treatment and control group design or a double pretest-posttest nonequivalent treatment and control group design. Single subject designs such as a treatment replication design or a multiple baseline across behaviors design also fall in the middle of most evidence models. Toward the lowest level of evidence are quantitative and qualitative descriptive case studies and correlation/regression research. Table 6–5 gives examples of levels of evidence and the corresponding research designs.

When using levels of evidence, such as those in Table 6–5, we should keep in mind that most of the published models are for evaluating intervention research; and the

---

[3]Those who are interested in the levels of evidence used in medicine and procedures for critical evaluation of research might consult Harbour and Miller (2001) and Phillips et al. (2001).

Table 6–5. Levels of evidence for intervention research commonly cited in the literature on evidence based practice and the related research designs

Levels of Evidence	Research Designs
Meta-analysis	• Combined analysis of several randomized clinical trials
Randomized Clinical Trial	• Posttest-only randomized groups designs • Pretest-posttest randomized groups designs • Solomon randomized four-group design • Randomized switching replications design • Randomized factorial designs
Nonrandomized Control Study	• Pretest-posttest nonequivalent groups designs • Switching replications design with nonequivalent groups • Double pretest-posttest nonequivalent groups designs
Other Quasi-Experimental Study	• Repeated measures experimental designs (with or without counterbalancing) • A_1-B-A_2 treatment withdrawal single-subject design • A_1-B_1-A_2-B_2 treatment replication single-subject design • A_1-B-A_2-C-A_3 multiple treatment single-subject design • Single-subject multiple baseline across behaviors design • Single-subject multiple baseline across participants design
Nonexperimental Studies	• Quantitative and qualitative descriptive case studies • Correlation and regression research • Comparisons of groups with preexisting characteristics • Qualitative research approaches including ethnography, grounded theory, and phenomenology
Expert Opinion	• In the absence of previous empirical research

levels of evidence for other clinical questions, such as those related to diagnosis and prognosis, would be different. Qualitative research approaches, which fall at a lower level of evidence in the intervention model, would be considered one of the best approaches for investigating some clinical questions, such as those related to how a speech, language, or hearing disorder affects the experiences of individuals (Health Sciences Information Service, 2007).

Summary

Experimental research designs are nearly always the best approach when the goal of a study is to establish a cause and effect relationship, such as between an intervention and improvement in the participants' behavior. All experimental designs share the feature of an experimental manipulation, and the strongest experimental designs, called true experimental designs, also have the feature of random assignment of participants to at least one treatment and one control group. True experimental designs include variations with random assignment of participants to groups, such as posttest-only designs, pretest-posttest designs, switching replications designs, and factorial designs. When random assignment of participants to groups is impractical, researchers sometimes use a quasi-experimental design and compare pre-existing groups. Quasi-experimental designs include variations that parallel the true experimental designs, except with nonrandom assignment of participants to groups. Some examples include a pretest-posttest non-equivalent control group design, switching replications design with nonequivalent control group, and a double pretest design with nonequivalent control group. Quasi-experimental designs also include times series or single participant designs with experimental manipulation of a treatment variable. Examples include treatment withdrawal, treatment replication, and multiple baseline designs.

In evidence-based practice investigations, research design is one of the key factors in determining the level of evidence a study provides. At the highest levels of evidence are true experimental designs, which are sometimes called randomized clinical trials, and meta-analyses. A meta-analysis is a study that involves a statistical analysis of the combined results of several randomized clinical trials. Quasi-experimental designs fall in the middle range of most levels of evidence models. Both quasi-experimental designs with nonequivalent treatment and control groups and single participant research designs have experimental manipulation of at least one independent variable, but neither has the feature of random assignment of participants to groups. When judging the level of evidence for intervention studies, nonexperimental designs such as descriptive case studies, correlation research, and qualitative designs fall at a relatively low level of evidence, and suggestions based on expert opinion with little or no supporting evidence are at the lowest level.

Review Questions

1. The purpose of _____ is to explore cause and effect relationships.

2. What are two important characteristics of a true experimental design?

3. Explain the following design notation:
   R   O   X   O
   R   O   O

4. What is the primary distinction between a true experimental design and a quasi-experimental design?

5. What is the design notation for a switching replications design?

6. Why is a switching replications design a good choice for intervention research?

7. Explain the concept of *pretest sensitization* (reactive effect of testing).

8. Identify each of the following statements as most likely to apply to single subject or group research designs.

a. _____ Participants experience both the treatment and control conditions.

b. _____ A good approach when participants respond in unique ways to the experimental intervention.

c. _____ Data is usually presented in graphs or tables for individual subjects and often no statistical analysis is completed.

d. _____ Researchers usually report the combined results for all participants.

9. Explain how maturation is a threat to the internal validity of a study and how including both randomized treatment and control groups addresses this threat.

10. Explain how a repeated measures design would be different from a pretest-posttest randomized control group design.

11. A researcher wished to use a factorial design to study the length/scheduling of treatment sessions (30-minute sessions four times per week and 1 hour sessions two times per week) as well as two different approaches to providing feedback (immediate feedback following every response versus delayed feedback following each set of five responses). The researcher recruited 36 subjects with articulation and phonological disorders for the study. Illustrate how the subjects would be randomly assigned to groups in this factorial design.

12. What does the term statistical regression mean and how could this phenomenon affect the results of an intervention study?

13. What is the best way to control for most threats to internal validity?

14. Explain the difference between a multiple baseline across behaviors single subject design and a multiple baseline across subjects single subject design.

15. In most levels of evidence models, what kind of evidence is at the highest level and what kind is at the lowest level?

16. How are a systematic review and meta-analysis different from the narrative review of literature that usually begins a research report?

Learning Activities

1. Read one or more of the following published reports on research that employ a true experimental design. Identify the experimental manipulation and describe how participants were randomly assigned to groups.

Almost, D., & Rosenbaum, P. (1998). Effectiveness of speech intervention for phonological disorders: A randomized controlled trial. *Developmental Medicine and Child Neurology, 40*(5), 319–325.

Chisolm, T. H., Abrams, H. B., & McArdle, R. (2004). Short- and long-term outcomes of adult audiological rehabilitation. *Ear and Hearing, 25*(5), 464–477.

Cohen, W., Hodson, A., O'Hare, A., Boyle, J., Durrani, T., McCartney, E., et al. (2005).

Effects of computer-based intervention through acoustically modified speech (Fast ForWord) in severe mixed receptive-expressive language impairment: Outcomes from a randomized controlled trial. *Journal of Speech, Language, and Hearing Research, 48,* 715–729.

Doesborgh, S. J., van de Sandt-Koenderman, M. W., Dippel, D. W., van Harskamp, F., Koudstaal, P. J., & Visch-Brink, E. G. (2003). Effects of semantic treatment on verbal communication and linguistic processing in aphasia after stroke: A randomized controlled trial. *Stroke, 35*(1), 141–146.

Ebbels, S. H., van der Lely, H. K., & Dockrell, J. E. (2007). Intervention for verb argument structure in children with persistent SLI: A randomized control trial. *Journal of Speech, Language, and Hearing Research, 50,* 1330–1349.

Harris, V., Onslow, M., Packman, A., Harrison, E., & Menzies, R. (2002). An experimental investigation of the impact of the Lidcombe Program on early stuttering. *Journal of Fluency Disorders, 27*(3), 203–213.

Hesketh, A., Dima, E., & Nelson, V. (2007). Teaching phoneme awareness to preliterate children with speech disorder: A randomized controlled trial. *International Journal of Language and Communication Disorders, 42,* 251–271.

Rvachew, S., Nowak, M., & Cloutier, G. (2004). Effect of phonemic perception training on the speech production and phonological awareness skills of children with expressive phonological delay. *American Journal of Speech-Language Pathology, 13,* 250–263.

Sapir, S., Spielman, J. L., Ramig, L. O., Story, B. H., & Fox, C. (2007). Effects of intensive voice treatment (the Lee Silverman Voice Treatment [LSVT]) on vowel articulation in dysarthric individuals with idiopathic Parkinson disease: Acoustic and perceptual findings. *Journal of Speech, Language, Hearing Research, 50,* 899–912.

van Kleeck, A., Vander Woude, J., & Hammett, L. (2006). Fostering literal and inferential language skills in Head Start preschoolers with language impairment using scripted book-sharing discussions. *American Journal of Speech-Language Pathology, 15,* 85–95.

2. Think of an independent variable you would like to investigate. Perhaps focus on an intervention from the field of audiology or speech-language pathology. Think about whether you would investigate this variable with a treatment and control group or with two or more levels of treatment. Which of the true experimental designs discussed in this chapter would be appropriate for investigating the variable you chose? What measures will you use for your pretest and/or posttest? How many participants will you need to recruit and how will you assign them to the different groups?

References

Almost, D., & Rosenbaum, P. (1998). Effectiveness of speech intervention for phonological disorders: A randomized controlled trial. *Developmental Medicine and Child Neurology, 40*(5), 319–325.

American Speech-Language-Hearing Association. (2004). *Evidence-based practice in communication disorders: An introduction* [Technical report]. Retrieved January 3, 2007, from http://www.asha.org/docs/html/TR2004-00001.html

Ballard, K. J., & Thompson, C. K. (1999). Treatment and generalization of complex sentence production in agrammatism. *Journal of Speech, Language, and Hearing Research, 42,* 690–707.

Barlow, D. H., & Hersen, M. (1984). *Single case experimental designs: Strategies for studying behavior change* (2nd ed.). New York: Pergamon Press.

Bernthal, J. E., & Bankson, N. W. (2003). *Articulation and phonological disorders* (5th ed.). Boston: Allyn and Bacon.

Centre for Evidence-Based Medicine. (n.d.). *Levels of evidence.* Retrieved February 15, 2008, from http://www.cebm.net/index.aspx?o=1025

Chapman, R. S., Sindberg, H., Bridge, C., Gigstead, K., & Hesketh, L. (2006). Effect of memory support and elicited production on fast mapping of new words by adolescents with Down syndrome. *Journal of Speech, Language, and Hearing Research, 49*, 3–15.

Cherry, R., & Rubinstein, A. (2006). Comparing monotic and diotic selective auditory attention abilities in children. *Language, Speech, and Hearing Services in Schools, 37*, 137–142.

Chisolm, T. H., Abrams, H. B., & McArdle, R. (2004). Short- and long-term outcomes of adult audiological rehabilitation. *Ear and Hearing, 25*(5), 464–477.

Cook, D. J., Mulrow, C. S., & Haynes, R. B. (1997). Systematic reviews: Synthesis of best evidence for clinical decisions [Electronic version]. *Annals of Internal Medicine, 126*(5), 376–380.

Doesborgh, S. J., van de Sandt-Koenderman, M. W., Dippel, D. W., van Harskamp, F., Koudstaal, P. J., & Visch-Brink, E. G. (2003). Effects of semantic treatment on verbal communication and linguistic processing in aphasia after stroke: A randomized controlled trial. *Stroke, 35*(1), 141–146.

Drew, R. L., & Thompson, C. K. (1999). Model-based semantic treatment for naming deficits in aphasia. *Journal of Speech, Language, and Hearing Research, 42*, 972–989.

Elman, R. J., & Bernstein-Ellis, E. (1999). The efficacy of group communication treatment in adults with chronic aphasia. *Journal of Speech, Language, and Hearing Research, 42*, 411–419.

Gallagher, T. M. (2002). Evidence-based practice: Applications to speech-language pathology. *Perspectives on Language Learning and Education, 9*(1), 2–5.

Goldstein, H., English, K., Shafer, K., & Kaczmarek, L. (1997). Interaction among preschoolers with and without disabilities: Effects of across-the-day peer intervention. *Journal of Speech, Language, and Hearing Research, 40*, 33–48.

Gordon-Salant, S., Fitzgibbons, P. J., & Friedman, S. A. (2007). Recognition of time-compressed and natural speech with selective temporal enhancements by young and elderly listeners. *Journal of Speech, Language, and Hearing Research, 50*, 1181–1193.

Hancock, K., Craig, A., McCready, C., McCaul, A., Costello, D., Campbell, K., et al. (1998). Two- to six-year controlled-trial stuttering outcomes for children and adolescents. *Journal of Speech, Language, and Hearing Research, 41*, 1242–1252.

Harbour, R., & Miller, J. (2001). A new system for grading recommendations in evidence based guidelines [Electronic version], *BMJ, 323*, 334–336.

Harris, V., Onslow, M., Packman, A., Harrison, E., & Menzies, R. (2002). An experimental investigation of the impact of the Lidcombe Program on early stuttering. *Journal of Fluency Disorders, 27*(3), 203–213.

Health Science Information Service. (2007, November 7). *Evidence based practice (EBP).* Retrieved January 14, 2008, from http://consortiumlibrary.org/hsis/researchaids/handouts/ebp.php

Hesketh, A., Dima, E., & Nelson, V. (2007). Teaching phoneme awareness to pre-literate children with speech disorder: A randomized controlled trial. *International Journal of Language and Communication Disorders, 42*, 251–271.

Ilgaz, H., & Aksu-Koc, A. (2005). Episodic development in preschool children's play-prompted and direct-elicited narratives. *Cognitive Development, 20*, 526–544.

Kashinath, S., Woods, J., & Goldstein, H. (2006). Enhancing generalized teaching strategy use in daily routines by parents of children with autism. *Journal of Speech, Language, and Hearing Research, 49*, 466–485.

Kearns, K. P. (1986). Flexibility of single-subject experimental designs: Part II. Design selection and arrangement of experimental phases. *Journal of Speech and Hearing Research, 51*, 204–214.

Kennedy, J. J. (1978). *An introduction to the design and analysis of experiments in education and psychology.* Washington, DC: University Press of America.

Kouri, T. A. (2005). Lexical training through modeling and elicitation procedures with late talkers who have specific language impairment and developmental delays. *Journal of Speech, Language, and Hearing Research, 48*, 157–171.

Kratochwill, T. R. (1992). Single-case research design and analysis: An overview. In T. R. Kratochwill & J. R. Level (Eds.), *Single-case research design and analysis: New directions for psychology and education* (pp. 1–14). Hillsdale, NJ: Lawrence Erlbaum Associates.

Leary, M. R. (2001). *Introduction to behavioral research methods.* Boston: Allyn and Bacon.

Max, L., & Onghena, P. (1999). Randomized and repeated measures designs for speech, language, and hearing research. *Journal of Speech, Language, and Hearing Research, 42*, 261–270.

McReynolds, L. V., & Kearns, K. P. (1983). *Single-subject experimental designs in communicative disorders.* Baltimore: University Park Press.

McReynolds, L. V., & Thompson, C. K. (1986). Flexibility of single-subject experimental designs: Part I. Review of the basics of single-subject designs. *Journal of Speech and Hearing Research, 51*, 194–203.

Mendel, L. L., Roberts, R. A., & Walton, J. H. (2003). Speech perception benefits from sound field FM amplification. *American Journal of Audiology, 12*(2), 114–124.

Palmer, C. V., Adams, S. W., Bourgeois, M., Durrant, J., & Rossi, M. (1999). Reduction in caregiver-identified problem behaviors in patients with Alzheimer disease post-hearing-aid fitting. *Journal of Speech, Language, and Hearing Research, 42*, 312–328.

Patten, M. L. (2007). *Understanding research methods: An overview of the essentials* (6th ed.). Glendale, CA: Pyrczak.

Phillips, B., Ball, C., Sackett, D., Badenoch, D., Straus, S., Haynes, B., & et al. (2001, May). *Oxford Centre for Evidence-based Medicine levels of evidence.* Retrieved August 25, 2008 o=1025

Richards, S. B., Taylor, R. L., Ramasamy, R., & Richards, R. Y. (1999). *Single subject research: Applications in educational and clinical settings.* San Diego, CA: Singular.

Rosenthal, R., & Rosnow, R. L. (2008). *Essentials of behavioral research: Methods and data analysis* (3rd ed.). New York: McGraw Hill.

Scherer, N. J. (1999). The speech and language status of toddlers with cleft lip and/or palate following early vocabulary intervention. *American Journal of Speech-Language Pathology, 8*, 81–93.

Schlosser, R. W. (2006). *Systematic reviews in evidence-based practice, research, and development* (Technical Brief No. 15). Retrieved February 15, 2008, from National Center for Dissemination of Disability Research Web site: http://www.ncddr.org/kt/products/focus/focus15/

Shearer, W. M. (1997). Experimental design and statistics in speech. In. W. J. Hardcastle & J. Laver (Eds.), *The handbook of phonetic sciences* (pp. 167–187). Oxford, UK: Blackwell.

Silverman, F. H. (1998). *Research design and evaluation in speech-language pathology and audiology: Asking and answering questions* (4th ed.). Englewood Cliffs, NJ: Prentice Hall.

Trochim, W. M. K., & Donnelly, J. P. (2007). *The research methods knowledge base* (3rd ed.). Mason, OH: Thomson Custom.

Weismer, S. E., Murray-Branch, J., & Miller, J. F. (1993). Comparison of two methods for promoting productive vocabulary in late talkers. *Journal of Speech and Hearing Research, 36*, 1037–1050.

Winslow, M., & Guitar, B. (1994). The effects of structured turn-taking on disfluencies: A case study. *Language, Speech, and Hearing Services in Schools, 25*, 251–257.

CHAPTER 7

Research Participants and Sampling

When planning a study, researchers usually have a group of persons in mind who are the focal point of the study. These groups can be quite large, such as all persons in the United States who are age 65 and older, or all children between the ages of 2 and 4; or the groups can be somewhat smaller, such as all persons between the ages of 45 and 65 with sensorineural hearing loss, 5-year-old children with specific language impairment, or adults between the ages of 18 and 25 with a traumatic brain injury. Even when a group is relatively small, studying everyone who is a member of the group is usually impractical. As an alternative, researchers try to identify a representative sample of individuals from the group to participate in their research. The strategies researchers use to select participants and criteria for obtaining a representative sample are topics covered in this chapter.

Populations and Samples

Ordinarily, researchers expect the findings from their studies to apply to a fairly large group of individuals and certainly to a larger group than actually participated in the study. Researchers use the term *population* to refer to all of the persons of interest for a particular study (Patten, 2007; Pyrczak, 2006). This population is defined in the planning phase of the study and all the members have one or more predetermined characteristics. For example, researchers might define the population of a study as all 4- and 5-year-old children who are bilingual Spanish-English speakers, all adults ages 45 to 65 who are native English speakers with no known medical conditions, or adults with a sensorineural hearing loss with an onset after age 50. Although the population of interest often is relatively large, this is not always the case. For example, audiologists and speech-language pathologists might conduct a study of the persons served in a particular speech-language-hearing center to determine how satisfied they were with the services provided. One of the criteria for establishing the population for a study is that all members have at least one characteristic in common.

The persons who actually participate in a study usually are a *sample* from a larger population. Sometimes authors refer to research participants as the subjects of a study. However, recent guidelines from the

American Psychological Association (APA, 2001; 2005) suggest authors should refer to their participants in a way that either describes who they are (e.g., the first grade children, the high school students, the parents, the teachers), or their role in the study (e.g., the participants, the listeners). One goal in identifying persons to participate in a study is to recruit a sample that represents the population well. This means all members of the population should have an equal chance of being recruited to participate (Patten, 2007). Researchers particularly try to avoid systematically excluding some members of the intended population when they identify participants. Let's consider the example of a research team that wants to recruit preschool children for a study. The team obtains the names and telephone numbers of potential volunteers by leaving a description of their study and a sign-up sheet at locations in their community frequented by parents and their children. They follow up by calling each of the families; however, because the researchers call between 9:00 A.M. and 5:00 P.M., they inadvertently exclude many families with working parents. This is an example in which some members of a population do not have an equal opportunity to take part in a study.

Trochim and Donnelly (2007) make a distinction between the intended population for a study and the "accessible" population (p. 37). The intended population includes all persons to whom the researchers want to apply their results, and the accessible population represents the group from which the researchers actually recruit their participants. One reason for the difference between the intended and actual populations could be geographic proximity. The researchers might want to apply their findings to all persons in the United States with a particular speech, language, or hearing disorder, but the accessible population might only include those persons who live near the research facility. The accessible population might be a good representation of the intended population but in some instances could be systematically different. For example, researchers in a university setting could have more families with highly educated parents than would be the case in the general population. Sometimes researchers address issues such as geographic proximity by developing cooperative projects with researchers in other locations.

On occasion, researchers conduct a study in which they gather information from an entire population. When researchers attempt to gather data from all members of a population, the study is called a *census* (Patten, 2007; Trochim & Donnelly, 2007). Perhaps the most familiar census is the U. S. Census that is conducted every decade by the United States Census Bureau (2000). Another example of a census would be research conducted on all members of a small population. Examples of these types of census studies would be research on persons served at a particular rehabilitation facility or on all first grade children in a particular school district.

When researchers study a sample from a large population, they still want to draw conclusions about the population as a whole. However, instead of knowing the characteristics of the population, as they would if they conducted a census, researchers make *inferences* about the population based on the data they gather from their sample. An inference is a conclusion we draw in an indirect way. When researchers develop conclusions about a population based on data from a sample, their conclusions about the population are indirect and not based on actual observations of the entire population. Furthermore, the accuracy of these conclusions depends on how well the sample represents the population.

Usually researchers want to study a population of persons, and the sample is a group of persons selected from that population. However, sometimes the population is defined in a different way, such as all first grade classrooms in the United States or all utterances produced by a particular child (Woods, Fletcher, & Hughes, 1986), and the units sampled will be different as well (e.g., a sample of first grade classrooms or a sample of utterances).

Often in group studies researchers report their findings as numerical summaries (Pyrczak, 2006). If these numbers come from observations on the entire population, they are called *parameters*. If these numbers come from observations on a sample, they are called *statistics*. In Chapter 8 and Chapter 9, we discuss how researchers use statistics to describe their findings and to make accurate inferences about the populations of interest in their investigations.

Sample Characteristics

As noted earlier, the most common approach to group research is to study a sample and to infer characteristics of the population as a whole from the results of the sample. The value of this kind of research depends on how well the sample represents the population of interest. Thus, researchers want to know about sample characteristics, such as what population a sample represents and whether the sample is biased or unbiased.

A sample is representative if the characteristics of the sample are a good match for the characteristics of the population. One aspect of this is to understand the actual population from which you draw your sample. Sometimes it is difficult if not impossible to access the intended population. Perhaps researchers want to recruit 4-year-old children to participate in a study. However, they do not have a readily available list of 4-year-olds and their parents.

Instead, they have access to 4-year-olds who attend preschool programs in the community. If the researchers draw their sample from the preschool programs, this sample might not be an ideal match for the general population of preschoolers.

In addition to concerns about differences between the intended and accessible populations, researchers also need to avoid bias in selecting a sample. An unbiased sample is one in which all members of a population have an equal opportunity of being selected, whereas a biased sample is one in which some members of a population have an unequal opportunity, or perhaps no opportunity, of being selected (Patten, 2007; Pyrczak, 2006). One source of bias in sampling is *failing to identify all members* of a population (Patten, 2007), either because of differences in the accessible and intended populations or because the researchers used a sampling method that introduced a bias. For example, researchers might issue a call for participants in an ad in a newspaper and in fliers distributed throughout the community. If they select as their participants the first 50 persons who respond, it would be a biased way of selecting a sample. Persons who respond quickly to such an ad could be systematically different from those who take more time to respond.

Another source of bias is using a *sample of convenience*. This refers to using a group of participants who are easy to access (Pyrczak, 2006). A common example is research with college students, and particularly research with students in introductory psychology courses. University professors often conduct research in their areas of professional interest, and if young adults are an appropriate population for the research, students in introductory courses are a readily available source of participants. Some professors might offer credit toward the course grade to students who volunteer for their research. However, from an ethical standpoint professors should not require participation in research, nor should they offer such opportunities as the only way to earn extra credit.

Sometimes researchers recruit participants from existing community programs because contacting persons through these programs is less of an invasion of privacy. For example, researchers might make initial contact with a group of persons age 65 and older through a community activity center. The initial contact could be low key, perhaps through a flier distributed at the community center, and potential participants could provide their contact information voluntarily without undue pressure. However, a sample recruited in this way might not be representative of the general population of persons age 65 and older. One might speculate that persons who attend the community programs might be more outgoing socially or in better general health than those who do not attend. If researchers wanted to apply their findings to all persons in this age group, they would need to develop ways to contact and sample from all members of the population of interest.

Another reason a sample could be biased is through *volunteerism*. This is a source of bias that cannot be avoided, because the process of informed consent specifies that all persons who participate in research should do so on a voluntary basis. However, persons who volunteer to participate in research might differ from the general population in some systematic way. They might have a special interest in the topic of the research because of their own or a family member's experiences. They might have greater interest than usual in research because they have conducted studies of their own. These are just a few of the many ways research volunteers could differ from the overall population. To address this issue, researchers sometimes resort to incentives to increase the number who agree to participate, such as payments, extra credit points, and so forth.

Sampling Methods

Although certain types of problems in selecting a sample are difficult to avoid, particularly volunteerism, researchers prefer random sampling methods when they want to avoid systematic biases in choosing research participants. In this section, we cover some of the most common sampling methods.

Simple Random Sampling

The procedure researchers usually use to obtain an unbiased sample is *simple random sampling*. An important feature of this sampling approach is that every member of a population has an equal chance of being selected for the study (Patten, 2007; Pyrczak, 2006; Trochim & Donnelly, 2007). Theoretically, you could generate a random sample by writing participant identifiers on separate pieces of paper, placing them all in a hat, and drawing them out one at a time until you have the target number of participants. However, researchers often use random numbers to choose participants. One approach is to assign all participants an identifying number. The researchers might start with a list of potential participants, for example, a list of 100 volunteers. Each person on the list is assigned a three-digit number from 101 to 200, and then the researchers could consult a table of random numbers and select participants in the order their numbers appear in the table. Example 1 is a series of random numbers representing the first 10 participants.

Example 1

154, 196, 191, 108, 157, 143, 188, 152, 183, 140

Another way to use random numbers to select a sample is to use the random number function in a spreadsheet program. First, you would list all possible participants in one column of a spreadsheet. Next, you would use the random number function to generate a random number for each participant in a second column, and then you would sort the participants using the random number column as the basis of your sort. Look at Table 7–1 for an example of this approach. The first column shows the potential participants listed by their participant identifier. The second column shows the random numbers generated for each participant. The last two columns show the participants and numbers after they were sorted. If the researchers in this example wanted a sample of 15 participants, they simply would take the first 15 persons in the sorted list (e.g., QQ through NN). This example only includes 26 possible participants, but the list often would be much longer.

Systematic Sampling

Another approach that generally yields a sample that is free from intentional bias is *systematic sampling*. In systematic sampling you start with a list of potential participants, establish a sampling interval, and then select every so many participants according to the number representing your sampling interval (Patten, 2007; Pyrczak, 2006; Trochim & Donnelly, 2007). To illustrate, let's consider the case of a group of researchers who have a list of 2500 potential participants. They want to select a sample of 125 actual participants from this list.

To determine the sampling interval, they divide 2500 by 125, resulting in a sampling interval of 20. This means that the researchers will choose every 20th person from their list. Often, researchers using systematic sampling establish their starting point with a random number. For example, these researchers might have determined at random that participant 110 would be the first selected. They would start at 110 and continue through their list choosing every 20th person until they have a sample of 125 persons (110, 130, 150, 170, 190).

Stratified Random Sampling

When researchers want to increase the likelihood that their sample accurately represents the population of interest, they might use a strategy called stratified random sampling. In this approach researchers identify one or more criteria or *strata* that characterize the population of interest. Examples include the percentage of men and women in the population, the distribution of persons by age group, family income levels, parent education levels, and whether the person lives in an urban, suburban, or rural area. Often, the goal is to include a similar percentage of persons in the sample as was present in the population. For example, if the population percentages were 60% women and 40% men, and researchers want to match these percentages in a 125 person sample, they would include 75 women and 50 men. Speech-language pathology is an example of a field where including an equal number of men and women in a sample would not be representative of the population. Occasionally, the goal in stratified random sampling is to select an equal number of participants across the levels of a stratum. This is often true with sampling across age levels.

Table 7–1. Illustration of the use of a spreadsheet to generate a randomized list of research participants

Participant Identifier	Random Numbers	Sorted Participants	Sorted Numbers
AA	87	QQ	10
BB	21	GG	11
CC	71	EE	14
DD	83	HH	18
EE	14	BB	21
FF	43	PP	23
GG	11	XX	26
HH	18	RR	29
II	40	JJ	32
JJ	32	UU	36
KK	52	YY	37
LL	99	II	40
MM	42	MM	42
NN	47	FF	43
OO	79	NN	47
PP	23	KK	52
QQ	10	ZZ	53
RR	29	VV	59
SS	60	SS	60
TT	61	TT	61
UU	36	CC	71
VV	59	OO	79
WW	97	DD	83
XX	26	AA	87
YY	37	WW	97
ZZ	53	LL	99

Variations on stratified random sampling are often employed in generating samples for test norms (e.g., Dunn & Dunn, 2007; Goldman & Fristoe, 2000; Newcomer & Hammill, 1997; Reynolds & Bigler, 1994; Zimmerman, Steiner, & Pond, 2002) and less frequently in research reports (e.g., Smit, Hand, Freilinger, Bernthal, & Bird, 1990; Trulove & Fitch, 1998; Wilson, Beckett, Bennett, Albert, & Evans, 1999). Usually the goal of stratified sampling is not to make comparisons across the subgroups but to generate a sample that represents the diversity present in the population of interest.

Cluster Sampling

One additional sampling approach that yields a random sample is *cluster sampling*. In this sampling approach researchers begin by obtaining a random sample of predefined groups such as medical centers, classrooms, or communities. An example would be a random sample of all the kindergarten classrooms in a particular state. Sometimes cluster sampling is combined with simple random sampling in a procedure called *multistage sampling* (Patten, 2007). In this procedure, researchers begin with a random sample from the previously identified clusters. They could start with a list such as a list of all communities in the United States with a population greater than 100,000, or a list of all universities that offer audiology and/or speech-language pathology graduate programs. Then they would select a certain number of clusters at random from this list. Perhaps they could use random numbers to select 50 communities or 50 high schools. After selecting communities or high schools to investigate, the researchers could follow up by selecting actual participants from each high school or community using simple random sampling.

Patten (2007) noted that predefined groups or clusters tend to be more similar to one another than the population as a whole. Therefore, researchers usually use cluster sampling in studies with relatively large numbers of participants. Such studies often include many clusters so that no single cluster will overly influence the research results. Tomblin et al. (1997) conducted a study in which they used a variation on

cluster sampling, stratified cluster sampling. The clusters in this example were kindergarten children in previously identified elementary schools. The strata were schools classified as being in urban, suburban, and rural areas. These researchers sampled elementary schools or clusters from a group of urban, suburban, and rural schools, and then completed their research by testing the kindergarten children from each school who were eligible for the study.

The various options for random sampling are regarded as the best way to obtain a sample that is free from systematic bias. However, that does not mean that all random samples represent their populations well. On occasion researchers obtain a sample that either overrepresents or underrepresents some aspect of the population. For example, the population might include fairly equal percentages of men and women, but after random sampling researchers could end up with a sample that has 60% women and 40% men; or perhaps the researchers end up with a sample that include a disproportionate percentage of children with college-educated parents compared to those whose parents have a high school education. When these kinds of variances occur by chance, and not through some bias in the sampling method, the errors that occur are less damaging than systematic errors such as failing to identify all members of a population or using a sample of convenience (Patten, 2007).

Purposive Sampling

In some research the goal is not to generalize findings to a larger population but rather to obtain an expert opinion or the perspectives of persons who have had a unique experience. Researchers use *purposive sampling* when they need to recruit participants they think will be the best source of information for a particular issue (Patten, 2007). Professional expertise could encompass many areas of audiology, speech-language pathology, as well as speech, language, and hearing science. Perhaps researchers are interested in studying recommendations for feeding infants with a palatal cleft, services provided by speech-language pathologists in neonatal intensive care units, or industrial audiology services provided to a specific industry. The number of professionals who could provide meaningful information on topics such as these might be relatively small, and researchers would need to make a special effort to identify and recruit them as participants.

Qualitative researchers often are interested in studying persons or organizations that have had unique experiences and may employ purposive sampling to find appropriate participants. For example, they might be interested in how persons in a clinical or medical center react to an experience such as implementation of new regulations, how persons who faced a sudden onset speech, language, or hearing impairment reacted and adjusted to the changes in their communication abilities, or how an adult who recently received a cochlear implant experienced the preparation for and follow-up to the surgery. When the answer to a research question requires input from special persons, researchers have to make a purposeful effort to identify those individuals.

Random Assignment

For some studies researchers have to divide the participants into two or more groups. This is the case in any true experiment with treatment and no treatment control groups or experimental and alternate treatment groups. The preferred method for generating groups is *random assignment* of participants to groups. Although both random assignment and random selection involve procedures such as a table of random numbers or the random number function of a spreadsheet, the two are different processes that serve different roles in research. The purpose of random selection is to identify a sample of individuals who will participate in the study from a larger population. The purpose of random assignment is to divide all the participants into different treatment groups. Sometimes in research, using random selection to choose participants is impractical (Woods, Fletcher, & Hughes, 1986). This could be the case in audiology and speech-language pathology if the research involves persons with very specific diagnostic characteristics. For example, speech-language pathologists might want to conduct intervention research with 4-year-old children who have a moderate-to-severe phonological disorder and age-appropriate expressive and receptive language, or audiologists might want to conduct research with persons with bilateral sensorineural hearing loss with an onset after age 40 with certain audiogram characteristics. The number of individuals who fit these descriptions might be relatively small, particularly if the researchers are limited to working with individuals who live relatively close to their research site. In situations like this you could begin with purposive sampling to identify as many individuals as possible that fit your criteria and were willing to participate in your study. After identifying your sample, you could use random assignment to divide the participants into different groups.

In the example in Table 7–2, the researchers identified 30 participants using purposive sampling. Each participant received a random number using the random number function in a spreadsheet program.

Table 7–2. Illustration of the use of a spreadsheet to generate two treatment groups using random assignment

Participant Identifier	Random Numbers	Sorted Participants	Sorted Numbers	Treatment Group
P01	271	P26	006	A
P02	231	P20	058	A
P03	489	P07	068	A
P04	420	P14	079	A
P05	091	P05	091	A
P06	289	P19	095	A
P07	068	P15	098	A
P08	329	P17	107	A
P09	311	P10	114	A
P10	114	P18	125	A
P11	421	P23	151	A
P12	373	P24	181	A
P13	188	P13	188	A
P14	079	P28	194	A
P15	098	P30	198	A
P16	434	P02	231	B
P17	107	P21	245	B
P18	125	P22	251	B
P19	095	P01	271	B
P20	058	P06	289	B
P21	245	P09	311	B
P22	251	P29	317	B
P23	151	P08	329	B
P24	181	P12	373	B
P25	454	P27	386	B
P26	006	P04	420	B
P27	386	P11	421	B
P28	194	P16	434	B
P29	317	P25	454	B
P30	198	P03	489	B

The researchers sorted the list using the random numbers and then assigned the first 15 participants in the random list to treatment group A and the next 15 to treatment group B. This procedure would yield two treatment groups created at random that should be free of any systematic bias in the assignment of participants.

Sample Size

One additional thing to consider about the sample is the number of participants to include. In some types of research, such as single subject designs or qualitative case studies, a single participant might be adequate. However, having a sample that is too small could affect the validity of the conclusions obtained from group studies. Even with random sampling methods researchers might end up with a sample that does not represent their population well, and this problem is more likely if the sample is very small. Pyrczak (2006) noted that increasing sample size should increase how well a sample represents a population, sometimes referred to as *sample precision*. On the other hand, increasing sample size does not decrease systematic bias. If researchers use a sample of convenience or fail to identify all members of a population, for example, increasing sample size does not reduce the bias associated with these sampling problems. Thus, researchers recruiting 4-year-old children from local preschool programs will fail to include children who do not attend preschool in their sample, and even doubling the size of the sample does not reduce this source of bias.

Several factors affect decisions about sample size. When conducting a study to estimate characteristics of a population, such as a typical level of performance on

some skill or the percentage of persons exhibiting a certain trait, these factors include the size of the population of interest, how variable the levels of performance are, and how frequent the trait is in the overall population (Patten, 2007; Pyrczak, 2006). If a population is small (e.g., 50 members), the best strategy is to recruit all or nearly all members as participants. For moderately sized populations (such as 1000 members), the recommended sample is approximately 28% or about 280 participants, and for larger populations (100,000 members), the recommended sample size is approximately 0.4% or about 400 participants (Patten, 2007). These sample size recommendations are not absolute and need to be modified to accommodate other factors such as population variability and high or low prevalence of the trait under study. Generally, the more variable a population is for a behavior, the larger the sample should be, and the rarer a particular trait, the larger the sample should be (Patten, 2007; Pyrczak, 2006).

When conducting a study to investigate the difference between groups, such as between treatment and control groups, the factors that affect decisions about sample size include how large the group differences might be, variability of scores on the outcome measures, and how certain researchers want to be about detecting group differences (Bland, 2000; Pyrczak, 2006). If a sample is too small, a study has a low probability of detecting a difference that actually occurs in the population.

Let's compare two hypothetical intervention studies. In this example, a group of researchers investigated two different language intervention approaches. Previous experience with the approaches suggested that intervention A was slightly superior to intervention B at the end of 3 weeks of treatment. The researchers expect participants receiving intervention A to score on average about 2 points higher than those receiving intervention B. Variability in performance would also be a factor, and in this example, the researchers expect 95% of the participants' scores to fall within ± 12 points. The researchers found they would need to recruit approximately 400 participants for each intervention group to be reasonably sure of detecting this small difference. The researchers realized that recruiting 800 participants who fit their criteria was impractical.[1] One solution the researchers considered was to extend the treatment time to 15 weeks. Their previous experience suggested that participants receiving intervention A would score on average about 5 points higher than those receiving intervention B after 15 weeks of treatment. Assuming the same amount of variability in participant scores, the researchers would only need to recruit approximately 25 to 30 participants for each intervention group to be reasonably sure of detecting this larger difference.

Let's also consider how differences in variability would affect sample size requirements. In the example above, the researchers needed 25 to 30 participants for each intervention group if the expected difference was approximately 5 points and variability was such that 95% of the participants' scores to fell within ± 12 points. How many participants would be needed if variability is greater and 95% of the participants' scores fall within ± 18 points? The answer is that sample size requirements would increase and the researchers might need to recruit as many as 65 participants for each group. Rosenthal and Rosnow (2008) noted that researchers need to attend to sample size requirements or run the risk of reaching conclusions that are inaccurate or invalid.

When researchers have too few participants, they are less likely to detect differences that would actually exist if they could study the entire population. Using a sample that is too small might lead researchers to discard a new intervention that actually could have improved professional practice.

A challenge in planning research is finding the information you need to make decisions about appropriate sample sizes. Conducting a pilot study is one of the best ways to determine how much difference to expect between groups or how variable participants will be on outcome measures. In a pilot study researchers recruit a small number of participants and employ their research design with those participants. Through this procedure they have an opportunity to identify any problems with their experimental procedures, determine how much change participants might make, and determine the amount of variability that occurs on their outcome measures. Although having data from a pilot study is extremely valuable in planning research, conducting one is not always feasible. As an alternative, Trochim and Donnelly (2007) suggest careful review of published research that employed procedures and/or outcome measures similar to the ones you plan to use. The previous research should provide some guidance regarding how much variability to expect in performance on outcome measures and how much change to expect after a certain amount of treatment.

In an ideal world, researchers would always be able to conduct studies with an adequate number of participants. However, with many of the populations served by audiologists and speech-language pathologists, recruiting a large sample for a study is

---

[1]These sample size estimates are based on Table 12.4 in Rosenthal and Rosnow (2008). The initial assumptions were that the outcome measure had a standard deviation (SD) of 6 and that this SD was the same for both intervention groups.

very challenging. Rather than settle for only a small chance of detecting differences that actually exist in a population, researchers in communication sciences and disorders might consider other ways to improve their research. As we saw in our first example above, even a relatively small sample would be adequate if the effect of a treatment is large. One way to increase the effectiveness of a treatment is to assure that it is executed in a precise and accurate way, such as through extensive training of the person(s) who will provide the treatment (Trochim & Donnelly, 2007). The second example above illustrated how variability in performance affected sample size requirements. Thus, another way to improve the likelihood that you will be able to detect important differences is to reduce the variability associated with your outcome measures (Trochim & Donnelly, 2007). If you have a choice of outcome measures, using the one with a high degree of reliability or measurement consistency is important. If you are using a self-constructed measure, ways to increase reliability include increasing the number of items or trials and possibly improving the instruction for those who administer and score the measure. More reliable outcome measures could reduce the amount of variability researchers sometimes consider noise in their data relative to the systematic differences associated with the experimental manipulations.

Summary

One aspect of planning research is to define the population or group of persons who are potential participants. If this population is relatively large, a second aspect of planning is to consider how to obtain a representative, unbiased sample from this population. An unbiased sample is one in which all members of a population have an equal chance of being selected. A biased sample comes about when some members of a population are systematically excluded, such as when researchers fail to recruit some segment of a population or when they rely on a sample of convenience. Generating a sample in a random way using methods such as simple random sampling, systematic sampling, or stratified random sampling generally is the best way to obtain samples that are free of systematic bias.

In the field of communication sciences and disorders, researchers often engage in extensive, purposeful recruiting just to generate a sample of sufficient size. Samples generated in this way are not random samples, but researchers still could use random assignment to divide the participants into groups. Participants might receive their group assignment based on a series of random numbers, and thus each participant has an equal opportunity of being included in the various experimental and control groups.

Determining an adequate sample size is an issue that sometimes receives too little emphasis in research planning. A sample that is sufficiently large generally represents the characteristics of a population better than a sample that is too small. Further, in intervention research larger samples are more likely to reveal differences associated with treatment and control groups than samples that are relatively small. The appropriate sample size for research is not an absolute number but rather a variable number determined by factors such as how large the population is, how variable the population is for the characteristics under study, how frequent the trait is in the overall population, how large group differences might be, and how certain researchers want to be about detecting differences (Bland, 2000; Pyrczak, 2006). If researchers use samples that are too small, their findings are less likely to provide a true picture of the population as a whole and less likely to reveal differences that actually occur in the population.

Review Questions

1. What term refers to all persons of interest to researchers when they conduct a study? What term refers to the group of persons who actually participate in a study?

2. If all members of a population have an equal chance of being selected to participate in a study, is the sample biased or unbiased?

3. What is one reason that the intended population for a study and the accessible population could be different?

4. How could each of the following sources of bias affect the findings from a study?
   a. Failing to identify all members of a population
   b. Sample of convenience
   c. Volunteerism

5. Explain the procedures a researcher would use for each of the following approaches to random sampling.
   a. Systematic sampling
   b. Simple random sampling
   c. Stratified random sampling
   d. Cluster sampling

6. Which of the sampling approaches in question 5 is often used in obtaining normative data for our clinical tests?

7. Explain the difference between random sampling and random assignment of subjects to groups.

8. Identify each of the following statements as true or false.
   a. You can reduce the potential errors from using a biased sample by selecting a very large sample.
   b. Generally speaking, a larger sample yields more precise results because the sample is more likely to be representative.

9. The following example illustrates the use of random numbers to select participants for a study. The potential participants, listed by identification letter in column one, each received a random number as shown in column two. If a researcher selected participants by random number from lowest to highest, who would be the first five participants selected?

Column 1	Column 2
AB	105
CD	170
EF	129
GH	141
IJ	187
KL	158
MN	177
OP	121
QR	106
ST	131

10. Assuming all other factors are equal, which of the follow would require a larger sample?
    a. A behavior with high variability or a behavior with low variability

b. A group difference of 10 points or a group difference of 20 points

c. A trait that occurs rarely or a trait that occurs frequently in a population

Learning Activities

1. Use random assignment to divide your classmates into small discussion groups. You might use a spreadsheet application for this task. Start by listing all students in one column, and then assign each student a random number in a second column using the random number function. Finally, sort the students using the random numbers as your sort key. Once you have a randomized list you can divide the class by grouping every three or every four students.

2. Read a published report on some form of group research. What was the intended population for the research and what was the accessible population? How did the researchers generate their sample?

References

American Psychological Association. (2001). *Publication manual of the American Psychological Association* (5th ed.). Washington, DC: Author.

American Psychological Association. (2005). *Concise rules of APA style.* Washington, DC: Author.

Bland, J. M. (2000). Sample size in guidelines trials. *Family Practice, 17,* S17–S20.

Coladarci, T., Cobb, C. D., Minium, E. W., & Clarke, R. B. (2008). *Fundamentals of statistical reasoning in education* (2nd ed.). Hoboken, NJ: John Wiley & Sons.

Dunn, L. M., & Dunn, D. M. (2007). *Peabody Picture Vocabulary Test: Manual* (4th ed.). Minneapolis, MN: NCS Pearson.

Goldman, R., & Fristoe, M. (2000). *Goldman Fristoe 2 Test of Articulation: Manual* (2nd ed.). Circle Pines, MN: American Guidance Service.

Newcomer, P. L., & Hammill, D. D. (1997). *Examiner's manual: Test of Language Development—Primary* (3rd ed.). Austin, TX: Pro-Ed.

Patten, M. L. (2007). *Understanding research methods: An overview of the essentials* (6th ed.). Glendale, CA: Pyrczak.

Pyrczak, F. (2006). *Making sense of statistics: A conceptual overview* (4th ed.). Glendale, CA: Pyrczak.

Reynolds, C. R., & Bigler, E. D. (1994). *Test of Memory and Learning: Examiner's manual.* Austin, TX: Pro-Ed.

Rosenthal, R., & Rosnow, R. L. (2008). *Essentials of behavioral research: Methods and data analysis* (3rd ed.). New York: McGraw Hill.

Smit, A. B., Hand, L., Freilinger, J. J., Bernthal, J. E., & Bird, A. (1990). The Iowa articulation norms project and its Nebraska replication. *Journal of Speech and Hearing Disorders, 55,* 779–798.

Tomblin, J. B., Records, N. L., Buckwalter, P., Zhang, X., Smith, E., & O'Brien, M. (1997). Prevalence of specific language impairment in kindergarten children. *Journal of Speech, Language, and Hearing Research, 40,* 1245–1260.

Trochim, W. M. K., & Donnelly, J. P. (2007). *The research methods knowledge base* (3rd ed.). Mason, OH: Thomson Custom.

Trulove, B. B., & Fitch, J. L. (1998). Accountability measures employed by speech-language pathologists in private practice. *American Journal of Speech-Language Pathology, 7,* 75–80.

United States Census Bureau. (2000). *United States Census 2000.* Retrieved February 10, 2008, from http://www.census.gov/main/www/cen2000.html

Wilson, R. S., Beckett, L. A., Bennett, D. A., Albert, M. S., & Evans, D. A. (1999). Change in cognitive function in older persons from a community population: Relation to age and Alzheimer disease. *Archives of Neurology, 56,* 1274–1279.

Woods, A., Fletcher, P., & Hughes, A. (1986). *Statistics in language studies.* Cambridge, UK: Cambridge University Press.

Zimmerman, I. L., Steiner, V. G., & Pond, R. E. (2002). *Preschool Language Scale: Examiner's manual* (4th ed.). San Antonio, TX: Psychological Corporation.

CHAPTER 8

Data Analysis: Describing Different Types of Data

Once researchers have the information they planned to gather from their participants, the next phase of scientific inquiry is to organize and analyze that information. The information or data obtained from research takes many forms.[1] In previous chapters we discussed the basic distinction between qualitative, verbal forms of data and quantitative, numerical forms. Even for quantitative data the numerical information could represent one of several levels of measurement, and these different levels of measurement go with various procedures for describing and analyzing data. Thus, before beginning an analysis, researchers need to consider the nature of their measures and what analysis tools are the best match for those measures.

Levels of Measurement

Level of measurement refers to the nature of the numbers associated with a particular set of observations. Any phenomenon could be measured in several different ways. Let's consider the example of a speech sound.

Researchers could record several forms of information about a speech sound, including phonetically transcribing the sound, judging the degree of nasality present during production of the sound, counting the number of correct productions of the sound in a list of spoken words, obtaining an ultrasound image during production of the sound, measuring electrical activity in selected muscles using electromyography (EMG), obtaining duration, intensity, and frequency measurements from a spectrogram, or measuring oral and nasal airflow during production of the sound. These procedures could yield various types of numbers including frequency counts, ratings on a scale from 1 to 5, accuracy scores, or even proportions that reflect direct comparisons such as between oral and nasal airflow. These different types of data correspond to the different levels of measurement usually identified in most introductory statistics books. The field of statistics usually distinguishes four levels of measurement, nominal, ordinal, interval, and ratio, each with its own defining characteristics (Patten, 2007; Pyrczak, 2006; Trochim & Donnelly, 2007).

---

[1]When using the word *data* in your writing, keep in mind that it is a plural form. The singular form is the word *datum*.

The *nominal* level of measurement is sometimes referred to as the naming level (Trochim & Donnelly, 2007). When using a nominal level of measurement, researchers assign participants and their responses to categories such as male or female, type of utterance, type of audiogram, type of aphasia or other disorder, dialect of American English, and so forth. Nominal level measures are not ordered, and being assigned to a particular category is not necessarily better or worse than being assigned to some other category. In analyzing nominal data researchers could count the number of participants or behaviors that fit into a particular category, compare participants or behaviors by discussing if they are members of the same or different categories, and discuss which categories have the most or fewest members. However, they would not compare categories directly by suggesting a particular label is greater or less than or better or worse than another label.

Well-constructed nominal measures have categories that are exhaustive and mutually exclusive (Peers, 1996). Categories are exhaustive if every participant or every behavior under observation fits into a category. Categories are mutually exclusive if each participant or instance of a behavior fits into only one category. Researchers might use strategies such as adding an "other" category and combining characteristics such as expressive and receptive language impairment or mixed sensorineural and conductive hearing loss to assure having a set of categories that are both exhaustive and mutually exclusive.

The *ordinal* level of measurement corresponds to rank ordered data (Trochim & Donnelly, 2007). Either researchers rank participants and observations from high to low relative to one another, or researchers use a rating scale to assign an ordinal measurement to a series of observations (e.g.,

ratings from 1 to 5). With ordinal level measurement you know the relative positions of an observation or participant relative to others, but ordinal level measurement does not provide information about the amount of difference (Pyrczak, 2006). In comparing ordinal measures, you can discuss who ranked higher or lower on a particular trait, but you cannot equate differences in ranks. Thus, the difference between a rank of 3 versus 4 is not necessarily the same degree of difference as a rank of 5 versus 6. Let's say a researcher ranked a group of 10 preschool children on talkativeness during a 30-minute play session. The degree of difference between the child ranked 3 and the one ranked 4 could be unlike the degree of difference between the child ranked 5 and the one ranked 6. In one case the difference could be quite small, but in the other case fairly large.

Although ordinal measures often involve assigning numbers, using labels that represent relative traits is another possibility (e.g., mild, moderate, severe; poor, fair, good, very good, excellent; strongly disagree, moderately disagree, undecided, moderately agree, strongly agree). Further, having a low rank might be desirable or undesirable. For some attributes or events, it might be better to be ranked lower; for other attributes it might be better to be ranked higher. For example, a rank of 2 would be more desirable than a rank of 5 if the scale of measurement was a severity rating scale where a 1 corresponded to a mild impairment and 5 corresponded to a severe impairment. However, the reverse would be true if the scale of measurement was an intelligibility rating scale where a 1 corresponded to always unintelligible and 5 corresponded to always intelligible.

The *interval* level of measurement provides information about which participants have higher or lower scores, as well as by *how much* participants differ (Trochim & Donnelly, 2007). To interpret "how much" you need a measure that yields equal intervals. This means that the difference between scores of 25 and 35 is the same amount as the difference between scores of 50 and 60. Let's revisit the example of the researcher who studied the talkativeness of 10 preschool children. Instead of ranking the children on talkativeness, the researcher might have used a more direct measure such as the number of words produced during 30 minutes of play. If the child ranked 3 produced 25 words and the child ranked 4 produced 35 words, whereas the child ranked 5 produced 50 words and the one ranked 6 produced 60 words, then we would know the amount of difference was the same (10 words).

The numbers on an interval scale can be added, subtracted, multiplied, and divided in a meaningful way without affecting the comparable intervals between numbers. For example, if we had a series of numbers that differed by 5 points, such as 20, 25, 30, 35, 40, 45, and 50, we could add 10 points to each number and the difference would still be 5 points: 30, 35, 40, 45, 50, 55, and 60. If we multiplied each number by 2 (40, 50, 60, 70, 80, 90, and 100), the interval between numbers would also double but would still be comparable. One characteristic that is lacking in interval level measurement is the ability to compare numbers directly. In comparing two interval level scores, such as 25 and 50, you could say the scores differ by 25 points, but not that a score of 50 is twice as good as a score of 25. This type of direct comparison, expressed in a proportion or quotient, requires a level of measurement with a true zero, a characteristic that is absent in interval level measures.

Many behavioral measures such as achievement tests, aptitude tests, expressive and receptive language tests, and percep-tual tests are interval level measures. Even when a participant receives a score of zero on such a test, it is difficult to claim that the participant has absolutely no ability on the skills assessed (a true zero). The participant might be able to score a few points if tested with other items and words that sample the same behaviors.

The *ratio* level of measurement has all of the features of interval level measurement, plus a true zero (Trochim & Donnelly, 2007). Ratio level measurements have three characteristics: (a) the ability to arrange numbers on a continuum, (b) the ability to specify amount and differences between amounts, and (c) the ability to identify an absolute zero relative to a characteristic. Thus, the difference between 20 and 30 is the same as the difference between 55 and 65. Further, a score of 60 would represent twice as much of the characteristic as a score of 30. Often, ratio level measures are assessments of physical attributes such as intensity, duration, or frequency measurements, electrophysiological measurements such as in EMG and auditory brainstem response (ABR) testing, or airflow measurements.

With knowledge of the level of measurement, researchers can make decisions about the most appropriate ways to represent and analyze their data. Some of these options include visual representations and descriptive statistics and are covered in the following sections.

Visual Representation of Data

One way to visually represent numerical information is to arrange it in a *table*. Research reports often include tables to convey information about participants, as well as the statistical findings of the study. The example in Table 8–1 illustrates a common

Table 8–1. Illustration of the use of a table to present participant information including participant identifier, age in months, and test scores

Identifier	Age	Test Scores Percentile Rank	Test Scores Standard Score
AB	48	9	80
CD	52	2	70
EF	46	2	68
GH	54	5	75
IJ	50	8	79
KL	46	5	76
MN	51	7	78
OP	45	6	77
QR	47	5	75
ST	53	10	81

way of representing participant information in a table. Publication manuals, such as the one from the American Psychological Association (APA, 2001), provide guidelines for how to organize and format tables.

Charts and graphs are ways to visually represent numerical information. These come in several forms and are useful either as supplements to information presented in tabular or text form or as the primary means of presenting data. Charts and graphs are particularly useful for live presentations and posters where numbers in a table could be difficult to read. Often graphs are the primary means of presenting and interpreting data in single subject design research (Franklin, Gorman, Beasley, & Allison, 1996; Parsonson & Baer, 1992; Richards, Taylor, Ramasamy, & Richards, 1999).

A type of chart that is appropriate for nominal, categorical measures is a *pie chart*.

Pie charts are useful for illustrating the percentages or proportions of observations that fit particular categories. You can use a pie chart if you have percentages or proportions that total to 100% or 1.0. An example of a pie chart is shown in Figure 8-1. This example figure shows hypothetical data from graduate students in communication sciences and disorders regarding where they plan to seek employment in the future. The size of a "slice of pie" corresponds to the percentage value. In the example the smallest slice corresponds to private practice (10%), and the largest slice corresponds to school (37%).

A *scatterplot* is another type of graph that is useful for illustrating the relationship between two, and even three, continuous measures. An XY scatterplot is a special graph that illustrates the relationship between two sets of scores, usually from the same participants. Scatterplots are useful for depicting relationships between measures, such as in correlation research. The example in Figure 8-2 illustrates a hypothetical study with 20 participants. This plot depicts a situation in which low scores on Test 1 correspond to low scores on Test 2, mid-range scores on Test 1 correspond to mid-range scores on Test 2, and high scores on Test 1 correspond to high scores on Test 2. The relationship depicted in Figure 8-2 also would be described as a linear relationship because the plot corresponds roughly to a straight line; however, scatterplots are not always linear, and some relationships might be nonlinear such as those shown by a U shape.

Column and bar graphs are useful for illustrating the magnitude or frequency of one or more variables. Researchers often use these types of graphs to depict group differences on measures such as frequency counts, percentages of occurrence, and

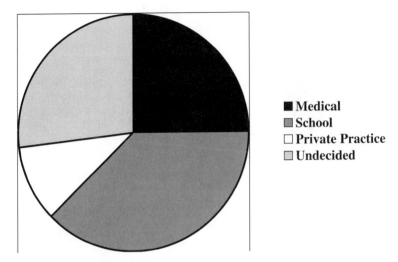

■ Medical
■ School
□ Private Practice
▨ Undecided

Figure 8–1. Illustration of the use of a pie chart to show nominal data by percentage.

XY Scatter Plot

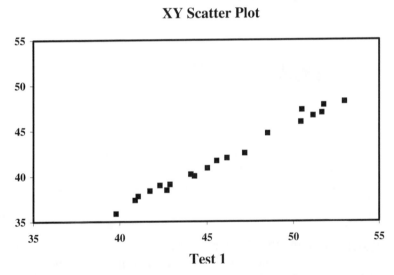

Test 1

Figure 8–2. Illustration of the use of an XY scatterplot to show the relationship between two continuous variables.

group means. Column and bar graphs are similar except for orientation of the display relative to the axes. In a column graph, as shown in Figure 8-3, columns originate from the horizontal axis and the height of the columns corresponds to the values for frequencies, means, and so forth. In a bar graph, as shown in Figure 8-4, bars originate from the vertical axis and the length of the bars corresponds to the different values.

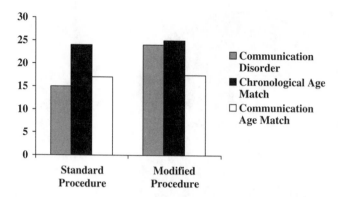

Figure 8–3. Illustration of the use of a column graph to show group means by experimental condition.

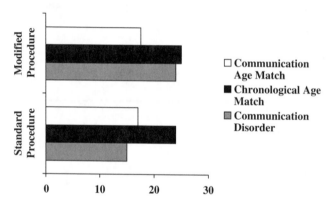

Figure 8–4. Illustration of the use of a bar graph to show group means by experimental condition.

One final type of graph that is common in research presentations and reports is a *line graph*. The functions of column, bar, and line graphs are similar because all three types are useful for illustrating different values for frequencies, counts, percentages, and averages. Depending on the nature of your data, these values could be associated with different groups, different tasks, different behaviors, changes over time, and so forth. Line graphs might be particularly suitable for depicting several values in a series or for depicting a special kind of nonlinear relationship called an interaction. An interaction occurs when two or more groups respond in unique ways to the experimental manipulations. The example line graph in Figure 8–5 illustrates an interaction in a simple 2-by-2 design, that is, a design with two different groups (e.g., persons with a hearing disorder or those with normal hearing) and two levels of the experimental manipulation (e.g., standard or modified test procedure). This example shows the use of a line graph to depict group means as well as variability within each group, as shown

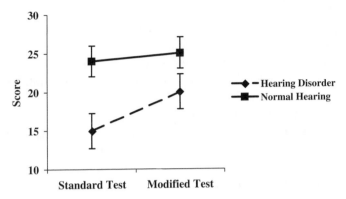

Figure 8–5. Illustration of the use of a line graph to show group means and standard deviations by experimental condition.

by the vertical lines extending from each mean.[2] By examining such a graph, you can readily see differences between the groups as well as differences associated with the experimental manipulation. Another characteristic to note in Figure 8-5 is that the lines representing each group are not parallel. The scores of persons with a hearing disorder improved more with the modified test (5 points higher) than the scores of the persons with normal hearing (1 point higher). This is what is meant by an interaction—the two groups responded to the change in test procedures in different ways, and these unique responses perhaps are easier to visualize with a line graph than with any other type of chart or graph.

Due to the greater cost of publishing graphic material as compared to textual information, researchers are fairly conservative about including charts and graphs in research reports. However, visual representation of data has a role in the initial stages of data analysis even if the graphs and

charts produced are not part of the final, published report. Further, visual representations are an essential part of live presentations and poster sessions, such as the ones you would see at local, state, national, and international conferences. The tools for generating charts and graphs are readily available in computer software you might already be using, such as spreadsheet and presentation programs.

Descriptive Statistics

Although charts and graphs provide an attractive way to display information, reporting data in numerical form is more common. Often the starting point in reporting results is to provide descriptive information about your data (Pyrczak, 2006). *Descriptive statistics* might be thought of as a way of summarizing data to convey the main information. Rather than presenting raw

---

[2]These vertical lines are sometimes referred to as *error bars* and often depict group variability by showing the mean ± one standard deviation.

scores, researchers present a few summary measures that capture the key characteristics of their data. Some of these key characteristics might include how often and how consistently particular behaviors occurred, what was typical or average among the participants or observations, and how variable behaviors were among participants.

Frequencies and Percentages

A frequency count or percentage could be the preferred descriptive measure when researchers want to convey how often particular phenomena occurred in a set of data. Frequencies and percentages are the primary descriptive statistics for nominal level measures. You might obtain a frequency count of the number of participants who fit a particular nominal category or the number of behaviors that fit a particular classification. For example, a university with

a graduate program in audiology might survey its recent graduates to determine their primary work setting. This example is shown in Table 8–2. The frequencies in this case represent the number of survey participants who reported working in each setting. The most frequently reported settings were hospital, physician's office, and health clinic or other nonresidential facility. The least frequently reported settings were school, university, and other.

Although research often involves classification of individual participants, sometimes frequency counts are based on a series of observations from the same participant. The data in Table 8–3 illustrate this possibility. In this example, a speech-language pathologist (SLP) was concerned about the behavior of a child who participated in small group treatment. The child exhibited frequent off-task behaviors and the SLP decided to document these behaviors before implementing an intervention to reduce

Table 8–2. Hypothetical results from a survey of audiologists who graduated from a university program in the last 5 years: Frequencies and percentages by work setting[1]

Work Setting	Frequency	Percentage
School	6	10
University	5	8
Hospital	16	27
Physician's office	16	27
Health clinic or other nonresidential	15	25
Other	2	3
Total	60	100

[1]These data are hypothetical, but the percentages are based on the 2006 American Speech-Language-Hearing Association Audiology Survey.

Table 8–3. Hypothetical results from a series of observations of a child's behavior during small group language activities

Behavior	Frequency	Percentage
On-task behavior	10	25
Fidget in chair	8	20
Talk/act while receiving an instruction	6	15
Talk/act during another child's turn	4	10
Prolonged look away from activity	6	15
Leave seat at inappropriate time	4	10
Other off-task	2	5
Total	40	100

their occurrence. The SLP videotaped two 30-minute group sessions and analyzed the middle 20 minutes of each session by classifying the child's behavior every 2 minutes. Thus, the SLP made 40 behavioral observations and classified these behaviors into seven categories, as shown in Table 8–3. The hypothetical data show that on-task behaviors occurred in 10 of the observations, and various off-task behaviors occurred in the other 30 observations. The most frequent off-task behavior was fidgeting.

A *percentage* (%) of occurrence is calculated by dividing the number of participants or observations in a particular category (i.e., the smaller number) by the total number across all categories (the larger number), and then multiplying the result by 100. Allowing for some minor differences associated with rounding, the percentages for each category should add to 100%. When reporting percentages, researchers usually include the raw numbers as well to clearly convey the nature of their data. Sample size is important for determining how well a set of observations might represent the population as a whole. A behavior that

occurs 2 times out of 10 and one that occurs 10 times out of 50 both occur 20% of the time, but a sample of 50 should be more representative than a sample of 10.

An alternative to a percentage is to calculate a *proportion*. Proportions and percentages yield related numbers. A proportion is calculated by dividing the number for a particular category by the total number, yielding a number between 0.0 and 1.0, because the number for a particular category could range from none to all. If you went one step further and multiplied by 100, you obtain a percentage, a number between 0 and 100. When using percentages you think of the construct under study as having multiple instances, such as 60 graduates of the audiology program (see Table 8–2) or 40 behavioral observations (see Table 8–3). When using proportions you think of the construct as a unitary phenomenon, such as one sample of recent graduates or one sample of behaviors. Thus, you could pose a question such as, "What percentage of graduates work in a hospital setting?" or, "What proportion of the sample works in a hospital setting?" Based on the data in Table 8–2, the answer to the first question would be 27%, and the answer to the second question would be 0.27.

When data involve information from participants or observations of a series of behaviors, researchers typically report frequencies and percentages. Conceptually, the notion of a proportion associated with persons, such as 0.27 audiologists, is awkward. However, some entities are easy to think of in proportions. For example, we might ask for a slice of pie that is one sixth or one eighth the size of the whole pie, corresponding to proportions of 0.167 and 0.125, respectively. As another example, we could think of a consonant sound, such as /z/, as a unitary construct. One could measure the duration of such a sound, perhaps finding that one such production in the word *buzz* had a duration of 250 milliseconds. Another characteristic of /z/ is that speakers tend to devoice this sound at the end of words (Small, 2005). Thus, we could ask a question such as, "What proportion of /z/ is devoiced when produced at the end of words?" If we analyzed a production and found the first 150 milliseconds was voiced and the final 100 milliseconds was devoiced, we could state that a proportion of 0.40 was devoiced (i.e., 100 divided by 250). Frequencies, percentages, and proportions are important ways of reporting nominal level data. However, frequency counts are useful in reporting other measures as well, such as the number of participants receiving a particular rating on an ordinal level scale or the number of participants receiving a certain score on an interval/ratio level measure.

Measures of Central Tendency

Measures of central tendency convey information about typical and usual responses of participants, or the score that falls toward the middle of a set of scores (Patten, 2007; Pyrczak, 2006). In everyday life we use the word *average* to refer to a typical person or response. Researchers identify specific ways to measure central tendency, and the three common ways are the mode, median, and mean. The *mode* is based on frequency information and is the category, response, or score that occurs most often. The mode is the only measure of central tendency for nominal measures; however, you can compute a mode for all levels of data, nominal, ordinal, interval, or ratio. First, let's consider the data in Table 8–3. In this example the mode, or most frequently occurring category, was "on-task behavior." For the data in Table 8–2, two categories were most frequent. Both "hospital" and "physician's office" had frequencies of 16 and this was the highest number in the set, so these data could be called *bimodal.* You can determine the mode for a set of interval/ratio level measures too, as illustrated in Example 1. In this set of numbers, a score of 75 occurs most often and is the mode.

Example 1

50, 55, 60, 65, 75, 75, 75, 80, 80, 85, 90

The mode is not always in the center of a set of scores, as illustrated in Example 2. In this series of numbers, a score of 55 occurs most often. Thus, the mode in Example 2 is 55, a number in the low end of the series.

Example 2

50, 55, 55, 55, 60, 65, 70, 70, 75, 80, 85

The *median* is a number that occurs at the midpoint in a series of scores. In publications, the abbreviation for median is *Mdn* (APA, 2001). To compute a median, you need numbers that can be ordered from low to high (or from high to low). Because of this, a median is appropriate for ordinal, interval, and ratio level measures but not appropriate for nominal level measures. If a series of scores represents an odd number of observations, calculating the median is straightforward. The median will be the middle score with an equal number of scores falling above it and below it. Example 2 above has a series of 11 scores. The middle score and median is 65, which has 5 scores above it and 5 scores below it. If a series of scores represents an even number of observations, determining the median is slightly more complex. First you identify the two middle scores that divide the series in half. Then, you use a process of interpolation to determine the number that falls halfway between the two middle scores. If a series of numbers has 10 scores, for example, the lower half will have 5 scores and the upper half will have 5 scores. The median will be the value that falls halfway between the 5th and 6th scores. Let's add a score to the series in Example 2 and create a series with 12 scores (see Example 3). In this example the middle two scores are 65 and 70, and the number that falls halfway between them is 67.5.

Example 3

50, 55, 55, 55, 60, 65, 70, 70, 75, 80, 85, 90

Identifying the median in a small set of scores is relatively easy. However, with a large set of scores, you might consider entering the data in a spreadsheet and using a statistical function for calculating medians or even using software designed specifically for statistical computations. If you have ever administered a test and determined the percentile rank for a client's raw score, you have used numbers that share a relationship with the median. If a client's score

fell at a percentile rank of 50, that score would be at the midpoint in the distribution, half of the scores falling above it and half falling below it.

The *mean* is a common measure of central tendency and when persons use the term "average," they usually are referring to a mean. The recommended publication abbreviation for mean is *M* (APA, 2001), although some statistical textbooks might still use an *X*-bar symbol. You compute a mean by summing all of the scores in a series and dividing by the total number of scores. The mean is most appropriate for data at the interval or ratio levels of measurement. In general, the mean is most reflective of data when the distribution of scores fits a normal distribution or close to it. If your data seriously violate a normal distribution, such as with extreme outliers, then you might consider a median rather than mean as your measure of central tendency. Example 4 includes two sets of data. In the first series, the mean and median are both 75. In the second series, one number was replaced with an outlier, an extremely low score. This extreme score impacted the value of the mean by lowering it to 70.9 but had no effect on the median.

Example 4

55, 60, 65, 70, 75, 75, 75, 80, 85, 90, 95
(*M* = 75.0 and *Mdn* = 75.0)

30, 55, 60, 65, 70, 75, 75, 80, 85, 90, 95
(*M* = 70.9 and *Mdn* = 75.0)

Calculating a mean may yield a number that never occurred in your data set. In the example above, all of the scores are whole numbers, but the mean is a decimal number. Similarly, one often reads statements such as, "The average number of students in graduate classes is 24.5," even though you cannot literally have half a person.

Measures of Variability

Usually, descriptions of a series of scores include measures of variability as well as measures of central tendency. Variability refers to the distribution or spread of scores around the midpoint of the scores (Pyrczak, 2006). As with measures of central tendency, researchers have many options for conveying the amount of variability in their data. The simplest way to convey variability is to report the *minimum and maximum* scores in a series. The scores in Example 4 illustrate one of the weaknesses of using this simple approach. In the first set of scores, the minimum value is 55 and the maximum is 95. The midpoint between these two scores is 75, which does correspond to the mean and median. However, in the second series the minimum is 30 and the maximum is 95. The midpoint between these scores is 60, which is much lower than the actual mean and median.

Another relatively simple measure of variability is the *range*. The calculation of a range utilizes the minimum and maximum scores in a series; however, we need to distinguish between reporting a true range and the actual minimum and maximum scores. An actual range, as defined by statisticians, is the *difference* between the highest and lowest scores. If the minimum value is 55 and the maximum is 95, the range is 40 (95 minus 55). In the field of communication sciences and disorders, researchers often report minimum and maximum scores using statements such as, "The scores ranged from 75 to 125." We need to keep in mind that the phrase "ranged from" is associated with reporting the lowest and highest scores and not the difference between these scores (125 – 75 or 50). Like minimum and maximum scores, a major disadvantage of the range is that a single extremely low or extremely high score could make a set of numbers appear more variable than they actually are.

When a set of scores has an extremely high or low value, an alternative to the range is an *interquartile range*. The interquartile range is similar to the range, except it represents the difference between the score that falls at the 75th percentile and the score that falls at the 25th percentile. Interquartile range characterizes the spread of scores in the middle 50% of your data. If 60 was the score that fell at the 75th percentile and 40 was the score that fell at the 25th percentile, then the interquartile range would be 20 (60 – 40 = 20). An interquartile range is a more stable measure of variability than the range because extreme scores have less impact on its value. However, computation and interpretation of an interquartile range is less straightforward than calculation of a range. For this reason, researchers are less likely to report interquartile ranges than other measures of variability.

When the level of measurement is interval or ratio, the most commonly used measure of variability is a *standard deviation*. The recommended publication abbreviation for standard deviation is *SD* (APA, 2001). The standard deviation reflects the dispersion of scores around the mean. Unlike the range, the calculation of a standard deviation uses all scores in the set; therefore, extreme scores have less influence on a standard deviation than a range (Pyrczak, 2006; Trochim & Donnelly, 2007). A larger standard deviation means you have a larger spread of scores around the mean. Thus, a set of scores that clusters close to the mean will have a relatively small standard deviation, and a set of scores that disperses widely from the mean will have a relatively large standard deviation.

Calculation of a standard deviation is fairly easy to understand. Usually, all scores are listed in a column as shown in Table 8–4.

Table 8–4. An example of the calculation of a standard deviation using a sample from a hypothetical set of data.

Raw Score	Raw Score Minus the Mean	Difference Squared
20	–31.2	973.44
30	–21.2	449.44
70	18.8	353.44
60	8.8	77.44
45	–6.2	38.44
60	8.8	77.44
60	8.8	77.44
35	–16.2	262.44
35	–16.2	262.44
45	–6.2	38.44
35	–16.2	262.44
45	–6.2	38.44
35	–16.2	262.44
70	18.8	353.44
30	–21.2	449.44
65	13.8	190.44
65	13.8	190.44
45	–6.2	38.44
50	–1.2	1.44
55	3.8	14.44
55	3.8	14.44
60	8.8	77.44
70	18.8	353.44
75	23.8	566.44
65	13.8	190.44
Mean = 51.2	Sum = 0.0	Sum of Squares = 5614.00
		Divided by n – 1 = 233.92 (Variance)
		Square Root = 15.29 (Standard Deviation)

First, you need to compute the mean for the set of scores. Then you obtain the difference between each score and the mean, as shown in the second column. If you simply summed these differences, however, the numbers would sum to zero with the differences above the mean canceling the differences below the mean. Therefore, the next step involves squaring the differences to eliminate the negative numbers as shown in the third column. At this point you sum the squared differences, yielding a value called the *sum of squares*. When you are working with a sample from a larger population, the next step is to divide the sum of squares by the number of participants minus one (n − 1). This value is referred to as the *variance*, and the standard deviation is the square root of the variance. Although calculation of a standard deviation is relatively clear-cut, the easiest way to obtain this value is to use the standard deviation statistical function that is available in most spreadsheet programs. Using a spreadsheet or statistical software for this calculation is particularly valuable when you are working with a large set of numbers.

Shapes of Distributions

Now that we have information about measures of central tendency and variability, we will consider one additional topic related to description of data. Certain measures such as the mean and standard deviation are easiest to interpret when scores disperse in a certain way, called a normal distribution.

Figure 8-6 illustrates a set of data that are roughly normally distributed. In a normal distribution, the dispersion of scores around the mean is symmetrical, and half of the scores fall above the mean and half fall below the mean. Further, the mean and median reflect the same value (50 in the example in Figure 8-6). Another characteristic of a normal distribution is that about 34% of the scores fall within one standard deviation below the mean and another 34% fall within one standard deviation above the mean. Thus, approximately 68% of the scores fall within ±1 standard deviation from the mean. If you consider two standard deviations above and below the mean, you would find approximately 95% of the scores fall within ±2 standard deviations from the mean.

Knowing how your data distribute from low to high around the mean is important because it helps you select appropriate descriptive and inferential statistics. Usually, selection of procedures for statistical analysis depends on the distribution of data in a population. However, researchers seldom have access to actual population parameters; the best alternate is to examine the distribution of scores in your sample (Coladarci, Cobb, Minium, & Clarke, 2008). A special type of graph, a *frequency polygon*, is a

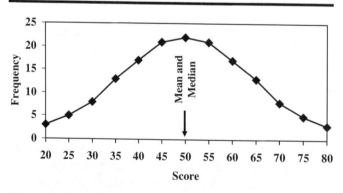

Figure 8–6. A frequency polygon illustrating a set of scores that are roughly normally distributed.

way to examine the shape of your distribution. The graph in Figure 8-6 is a frequency polygon, as are the examples in the figures that follow. To construct a frequency polygon, first determine how many persons achieved a certain score (e.g., how many had a score of 50, a score of 45, and so forth). Sometimes researchers group scores to construct the polygon by counting how many scores fell in a certain interval (e.g., how many fell from 46 to 50, from 41 to 45, and so forth). Once you determine the frequency of each score, you simply plot frequency on the vertical axis and scores on the horizontal axis using a graph such as a scatterplot with lines. After making your plot, you visually inspect the plot and decide whether or not the shape approximates that of a normal curve. Keep in mind that a distribution will not be very smooth unless you have a large sample. Figure 8-6 illustrates a distribution that is roughly normally distributed with a relatively wide spread of scores from 20 to 80. In contrast, Figure 8-7 illustrates a distribution that also is roughly normally distributed but with a relatively narrow spread of scores from 35 to 65.

Another way to think about generating a frequency polygon and inspecting the plot is that you are looking for the presence of scores that separate quite a bit from the other scores. These are sometimes called *outliers*. When a set of scores has outliers, the shape of the frequency polygon changes and the distribution no longer approximates a normal curve. Researchers often describe sets of scores with outliers as having a positive or negative skew. In a frequency polygon with a *positive skew*, the distribution has an abnormally long tail that stretches in the positive direction, as shown in Figure 8-8. The lengthened tail occurs when the set of scores includes a few that are higher than would be expected in a normal distribution. Another consequence, as we noted when discussing the computation of the mean and median, is that extreme positive scores pull the mean higher, producing a set of data in which the mean is higher than the median.

Outliers could occur in the opposite direction as well. In a frequency polygon with a *negative skew*, the distribution has an abnormally long tail that stretches in the negative direction, as shown in Figure 8-9. In this case, the lengthened tail occurs when the set of scores includes a few that are lower than would be expected in a normal distribution. These extreme negative scores

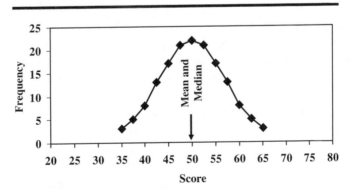

Figure 8–7. A frequency polygon illustrating a set of scores that are roughly normally distributed but have a relatively narrower spread and smaller standard deviation than the scores in Figure 8–6.

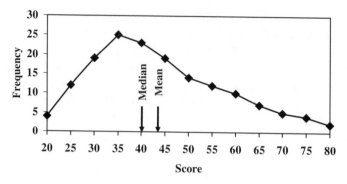

Figure 8–8. A frequency polygon illustrating a set of scores with a positive skew.

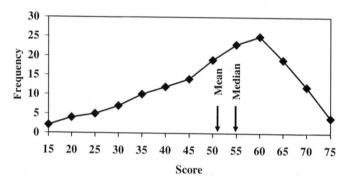

Figure 8–9. A frequency polygon illustrating a set of scores with a negative skew.

pull the mean lower, producing a set of data in which the mean is lower than the median, as shown in Figure 8-9.

When data are skewed, measures of central tendency and variability are more difficult to interpret (Pyrczak, 2006). A few extreme scores might create the illusion of a difference that does not really exist or even mask a true difference. Departures from a normal distribution are most likely with small sample sizes, and when working with small groups of participants, researchers need to be careful about their choice of statistical analysis procedures (Gibbons & Chakraborti, 2003; Woods, Fletcher, & Hughes, 1986).

Summary

One of the first steps in reporting research findings is to describe and summarize your findings. For quantitative data, researchers typically use descriptive statistics and/or visual displays, and the choice of appropriate procedures depends in part on the level of measurement for the outcome or dependent variables. The field of statistics usually distinguishes four levels of measurement, nominal, ordinal, interval, and ratio. The nominal level of measurement encompasses naming or categorizing observations, the ordinal level of measurement relates to placing observations in order or ranking them, and the interval level measures enable you to specify how much scores differ and not just which scores are higher or lower. Ratio level measures have all the characteristics of interval level measures and also have a true zero. Because of this, ratio level measures allow researchers to directly compare scores in proportional relationships.

Researchers have many options for the visual representation of data, ranging from numerical tables to various types of charts and graphs. The choice of visual display depends in part on your level of measurement and also on the nature of your research design. For example, a pie chart is a visual display that is appropriate for nominal measures that can be summarized with percentages or proportions. A scatterplot is useful in showing the relationship between two continuous measures, such as in correlation studies. Other options for visual displays include column, bar, and line graphs. These types of graphs are often used to display data from group comparison research.

Descriptive statistics are summary measures that convey the key characteristics of a data set. The options for describing data include frequency counts and percentages, measures of central tendency including the mode, median, and mean, and measures of variability such as the range and standard deviation. Each of these options fits certain types of data, and the challenge for researchers is to select descriptive statistics that are a good match to their outcome measures and research design.

One final consideration in describing your data is to determine how the scores distribute or spread around the center. Often, data fit a special kind of distribution called a normal distribution. Data that approximate a normal curve have a symmetrical distribution with roughly equal numbers of scores above and below the mean. However, data sometimes include extreme or outlying scores that alter the shape of the distribution. When a set of scores includes extreme outliers, the shape of the distribution is asymmetrical with an abnormally long tail in either the positive or negative direction. Outliers have a greater impact on certain descriptive statistics such as the mean and range, whereas other measures such as the median and standard deviation are more stable. Thus, the shape of the distribution, whether it is symmetrical or asymmetrical, has an impact on the researchers' decisions regarding what descriptive statistics to report.

Review Questions

1. Match the level of measurement with its brief description.

   _____ Nominal

   _____ Ordinal

   _____ Interval

   _____ Ratio

   a. Rank order from highest to lowest
   b. Shows how much participants differ, but no true 0
   c. Measures with a true 0
   d. Naming or mutually exclusive categories

2. Subjects in a study indicated where they live, which the researcher classified as rural/suburban/urban. What scale of measurement would this be?

3. Researchers classified preschool children's history of middle ear infections as frequent/moderate/ infrequent based on the number of reported episodes. What scale of measurement would this be?

4. The scores obtained from articulation/phonology or language tests most likely measure at what level?

5. What level of measurement would allow you to say that a score of 30 was three times as much as a score of 10?

6. What kind of chart or graph could you use if your level of measurement was nominal and you had percentages that totaled to 100%?

7. Explain when a researcher would use each of the following:
   a. Scatterplot
   b. Column graph
   c. Line graph

8. What descriptive statistics are used most often with nominal level measures?

9. Three measures of central tendency are the mode, median, and mean. What measure of central tendency provides information about the most frequently occurring category or score? What measure of central tendency is calculated by summing all the scores in a set and dividing that sum by the number of scores? What measure of central tendency provides information about the score that falls at the midpoint of a distribution?

10. What measure of variability is calculated by determining the difference between the minimum and maximum scores?

11. What is the relation between the standard deviation and variance?

12. Will an extreme, outlying score have a great impact on the range or the standard deviation of a set of scores?

13. What is the relationship between the mean and median in: (a) normal curve; (b) curve with a positive skew; and (c) curve with a negative skew?

14. Draw a distribution that illustrates data that approximate a normal curve, one that illustrates data with a positive skew, and one that illustrates data with a negative skew.

15. Draw the following:
   a. A roughly normal distribution with a mean of 50 and an SD of 5
   b. A roughly normal distribution with a mean of 50 and an SD of 10
   Try to use a similar scale of measurement in your drawings. Which distribution has the most variability?

Learning Activities

1. You have videorecorded a conversation between an adult with expressive aphasia and her spouse. Think of two examples of quantitative measures you could obtain from the speech sample and two qualitative descriptors you could use for the conversation. For your qualitative descriptors, try to use a precise level of description with minimal inference.

2. If you have access to a spreadsheet program, enter the sets of scores below into two columns. After entering the numbers, select the cell immediately below the first column, find the menu item for functions, and select the statistical function for average or mean. This should enable you to calculate the mean for the first set of data. Repeat this procedure for the second column of data. You can add the computation for standard deviation by selecting the menu item for functions and finding the standard deviation function. If your spreadsheet has a graphing function, you might try selecting both columns and generating a scatterplot for the two sets of scores. You also might try generating a column graph for the two means.

Set A	Set B
48	51
54	55
48	51
61	61
44	47
62	65
39	41
63	66
48	49
57	58
53	56
45	47
44	45
48	50
55	56
64	66
44	46
43	46
49	51
36	39

References

American Psychological Association. (2001). *Publication manual of the American Psychological Association* (5th ed.). Washington, DC: Author.

American Speech-Language-Hearing Association. (2006). *Audiology survey 2006: Clinical focus patterns.* Document retrieved March 18, 2008, from http://www.asha.org/NR/rdonlyres/5A8F29FE-47D8-4DCA-91F9-2094AD1E126F/0/06AudSurvey_focuspatterns.pdf

Coladarci, T., Cobb, C. D., Minium, E. W., & Clarke, R. B. (2008). *Fundamentals of statistical reasoning in education* (2nd ed.). Hoboken, NJ: John Wiley & Sons.

Franklin, R. D., Gorman, B. S., Beasley, T. M., & Allison, D. B. (1996). Graphical display and visual analysis. In R. D. Franklin, D. B. Allison, & B. S. Gorman (Eds.), *Design and analysis of single-case research* (pp. 119–158). Mahwah, NJ: Lawrence Erlbaum Associates.

Gibbons, J. D., & Chakraborti, S. (2003). *Nonparametric statistical inference* (4th ed.). Boca Raton, FL: CRC Press—Taylor & Francis Group.

Parsonson, B. S., & Baer, D. B. (1992). The visual analysis of data, and current research into the stimuli controlling it. In T. R. Kratochwill & J. R. Level (Eds.), *Single-case research design and analysis: New directions for psychology and education* (pp. 15–40). Hillsdale, NJ: Lawrence Erlbaum Associates.

Patten, M. L. (2007). *Understanding research methods: An overview of the essentials* (6th ed.). Glendale, CA: Pyrczak.

Peers, I. (1996). *Statistical analysis for education and psychology researchers: Tools for researchers in education and psychology.* New York: Routledge.

Pyrczak, F. (2006). *Making sense of statistics: A conceptual overview* (4th ed.). Glendale, CA: Pyrczak.

Richards, S. B., Taylor, R. L., Ramasamy, R., & Richards, R. Y. (1999). *Single subject research: Applications in educational and clinical settings.* San Diego, CA: Singular.

Small, L. H. (2005). *Fundamentals of phonetics: A practical guide for students* (2nd ed.). Boston: Pearson Education.

Trochim, W. M. K., & Donnelly, J. P. (2007). *The research methods knowledge base* (3rd ed.). Mason, OH: Thomson Custom.

Woods, A., Fletcher, P., & Hughes, A. (1986). *Statistics in language studies.* Cambridge, UK: Cambridge University Press.

CHAPTER 9

Data Analysis:
Inferential Statistics

In Chapter 8 we read about ways researchers might describe and summarize their data. A few summary measures that capture the key characteristics of the data frequently are more meaningful than the raw scores themselves. However, researchers often want to go beyond describing just the actual observations and want to develop answers that apply to a larger population. When researchers obtain information from a sample, one question they need to ask is whether their findings reflect the situation in the population in general, or whether the findings occurred because of some idiosyncrasy in the sample. Another way of phrasing this question is to ask what the chance or probability is that the findings from a sample represent the "true" situation in the population. Fortunately, the field of statistics provides researchers with tools for quantitative data analysis that allow them to draw meaningful conclusions about a population, even when they were only able to study a sample from that population.

Inferential Statistics

Once researchers have completed their observations and obtained a set of scores from their participants, they usually use some type of inferential statistical analysis to determine the likelihood that the findings from their sample represent the situation in the population as a whole. If the researchers could, hypothetically, study the population as a whole, would they obtain the same results? *Inferential statistics* is a tool that helps researchers test their findings to establish how representative they are. In a sense, one might think of inferential statistics as a tool for bridging from the actual observations of research participants to hypothetical observations of the population they represent. In generalizing from observations on a sample to the entire population the sample represents, researchers do not draw absolute conclusions. They do not make statements such as, "Our findings are or are not representative of the population in general." Rather, they make statements about how much *confidence* they have in their findings or about the *probability of error* associated with the results they reported. When you read a statement in a research report such as, "This difference was statistically significant," it means the researchers tested their data using some kind of inferential statistics and determined that the probability of error was acceptably low.

The need to submit research findings to a statistical test arises from the possibility of a sampling error (Patten, 2007; Pyrczak,

2006). Sampling errors occur inadvertently and can be present even in random samples from a population. Imagine that a researcher could draw 100 different random samples from a population. With that many samples, there is a possibility that at least a few samples have some peculiar characteristics and do not reflect the true nature of the population. If a researcher studied one of these unique samples, then the findings could reflect the unique characteristics of the sample rather the effects of an experimental manipulation. The role of inferential statistics is to provide information about the probability that the findings of a study were due to a sampling error rather than a true experimental difference (Pyrczak, 2006; Trochim & Donnelly, 2007).

In formal sense, inferential statistical tests are designed to determine the probability that a null hypothesis is true. Recall that a null hypothesis is a negative statement such as, "The experimental and control groups are not different" or "Scores from the experimental test and traditional test are not correlated." If the statistical test is significant, then the researcher will *reject the null hypothesis* because the probability it is true is quite low. Common levels for rejecting the null hypothesis are 0.05 or 5 in 100, 0.01 or 1 in 100, or the very conservative 0.001 or 1 in 1000. As we noted in the chapter on research questions, very few research reports include an actual statement of a null hypothesis or research hypothesis. Rather, researchers usually formulate questions or a statement of purpose to provide information about the intent of their study. Therefore, you will seldom read a formal statement about rejecting or failing to reject the null hypothesis. Researchers are more likely to conclude that they found a *statistically significant* result.

You might think of inferential statistics as providing information about the proba-

bility the findings of a study are in error, perhaps due to some sampling idiosyncrasy. Thus, if a statistic is significant at the 0.05 level, it means that the probability of error is less than 5 in 100. Similarly, a statistic that is significant at the 0.01 level means that the probability of error is less than 1 in 100. When researchers conclude that a difference is *not significant*, they have concluded that the probability of error in rejecting the null hypothesis is unacceptably high, usually because the chance of error is greater than 5 in 100.

Examples of things you might test with a significance test are associations or correlations, wherein the null hypothesis would be that there is "no relationship between the two variables," or differences, wherein the null hypothesis would be "no difference between the two groups." When researchers complete an inferential statistical analysis, they might report their findings with statements such as the examples below:

1. The null hypothesis was rejected at the 0.05 level.
2. The difference between means was statistically significant.
3. The difference between groups was significant at the 0.01 level.
4. The correlation between the two scores was significant at the 0.05 level.
5. The difference between groups was not significant at the 0.05 level.

One final concept to discuss is what researchers and statisticians mean when they talk about the possibility of making an error. Actually, researchers could make two types of errors when drawing conclusions about their data. The first kind of error is a *type I error*. This error occurs when a researcher rejects the null hypothesis when it is, in fact, a true hypothesis. In other words, the researchers concluded that two groups were significantly different when in fact the two groups were not different, or the researchers concluded that the correlation between two measures was significant, when the correlation was not actually significant. Inferential statistical tests are conservative and set up in such a way that the probability of making a type I error is kept very low (e.g., a 5 in 100 or 1 in 100 probability). Type I errors could occur because of sampling issues, when the participants in a study did not represent the general population very well.

The second kind of error is a *type II error*. This error occurs when a researcher fails to reject the null hypothesis when it is, in fact, an incorrect hypothesis. In other words, the researchers concluded that two groups were not significantly different when in fact the groups were different, or the researchers concluded that the correlation between two measures was not significant, when the correlation was actually significant. One reason that researchers might make a type II error is that the study lacked sufficient power. As we discussed in the chapter on sampling, the best way to increase statistical power is to recruit an appropriate number of participants. If increasing the number of participants is impractical, other ways to reduce the likelihood of making a type II error are to provide the experimental treatment and measure your outcomes in as precise and consistent a way as possible.

In the sections that follow, we are going to discuss two broad categories of inferential statistics, measures of association and difference tests. The notion that conclusions based on statistics are probabilistic rather than absolute applies to both categories of statistics. Researchers need to be equally careful about drawing erroneous conclusions whether they are investigating associations among different measures or investigating differences between groups.

Measures of Association

Researchers use measures of association when they are interested in investigating the relationship between two or more measures. For measures of association, each participant in a sample receives all of the tests or other observation procedures. If the researcher is comparing two different tests, then each participant completes both tests. Measures of association usually yield information about the strength of the relationship as well as the direction of the relationship (positive or negative) between measures. Some commonly used measures of association are correlation coefficients, such as the Pearson product-moment correlation coefficient and Spearman rank-ordered correlation coefficient. Other examples include chi-square analysis and contingency coefficients as well as simple regression and multiple regression.

Pearson Product-Moment Correlation Coefficient

If a researcher is investigating the relationship between two measures and the level of measurement is interval or ratio level, the most widely used measure of association is the *Pearson product-moment correlation coefficient*. The recommended symbol for the Pearson correlation coefficient is r (American Psychological Association [APA], 2001), and this measure of association is often called the Pearson r. The potential values of the Pearson r range from 0 to ±1.00 (plus or minus 1.00). A value of 0.00 would indicate that two sets of measures have no relationship, whereas a value of ±1.00 would indicate that two sets of measures have a perfect relationship (Pyrczak, 2006). The closer the correlation coefficient is to ±1.00, the stronger the relationship. The plus or minus indicates the direction of the relationship, but a *positive* correlation (e.g., +0.90) is just a strong as a *negative* correlation (e.g., −0.90). In some statistics textbooks the term *direct* relationship is used as a synonym for a positive relationship, and *inverse* relationship is used as a synonym for a negative relationship (Gibbons & Chakraborti, 2003; Patten, 2007; Pyrczak, 2006).

Perhaps the best way to understand the nature of the relationship expressed in a correlation coefficient is to produce a scatterplot of two measures and then compute the correlation coefficient. Figure 9–1 depicts the relationship between two variables that have a strong, positive correlation of $r = 0.98$. A few points to note about Figure 9–1 are that each participant completed both Test 1 and Test 2. The participants' scores on Test 1 are plotted on the vertical axis and Test 2 on the horizontal axis and each point corresponds to a participant. In this scatterplot, persons who obtain high scores on Test 1 also obtain high scores on Test 2, persons who obtain mid-range scores on Test 1 also obtain mid-range scores on Test 2, and persons who obtain low scores on Test 1 also obtain low scores on Test 2. Thus, the direction of the relationship is

positive or direct. Further, the relationship between the two tests is a strong one. The Pearson r is 0.98 and the scores tend to plot along a straight line with only small deviations away from the line.

Figure 9–2 illustrates a strong negative or inverse relationship between two variables. In this example, persons who score high on Test 1 score low on Test 2, whereas persons who score low on Test 1 score high on Test 2. Finally, Figure 9–3 illustrates a weak positive relationship between two variables. Note how the scores in this example scatter widely, approximating a wide oval shape. When the correlation between two variables is strong, the scatterplot approximates the shape of a straight line, and with a perfect correlation the scatterplot looks like a straight line. When the correlation approaches 0.00, the scatterplot approximates a circle (Coladarci, Cobb, Minium, & Clarke, 2008). Some authors have suggested verbal descriptors to use with different correlation values. For example, Patten (2007) suggested that a correlation of 0.25 was *weak*, 0.50 was *moderate*, and 0.75 and above was *strong*.

When interpreting a correlation coefficient, researchers consider the direction of

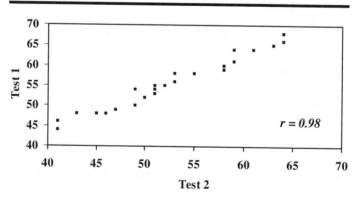

Figure 9–1. An XY scatterplot depicting the relationship between two variables with a strong, positive correlation.

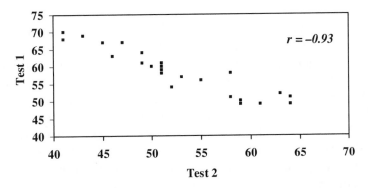

Figure 9–2. An XY scatterplot depicting the relationship between two variables with a strong, negative correlation.

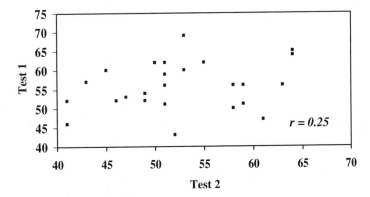

Figure 9–3. An XY scatterplot depicting the relationship between two variables with a weak, positive correlation.

the relationship, the magnitude of the correlation, and the possibility that the observed relationship between the variables occurred because of random chance. That is, researchers conduct a test of significance to determine the probability that the correlation between two variables represents the true situation in the population as a whole. If researchers found that a correlation was significant at the 0.05 level, they conclude that the probability the correlation occurred due to a random factor such as a sampling idiosyncrasy is less than 5 out of 100. Typically, researchers are comfortable with a 5% prob-

ability of a type I error (i.e., deciding that two variables were correlated, when they actually were not correlated in the general population). Plus, if researchers made their significance tests too stringent, they might increase the possibility of a type II error (concluding that two variables were not correlated when they actually were in the population as a whole).

Because the Pearson r is commonly used, most spreadsheet programs provide a function for calculating this statistic, as do most programs dedicated to statistical calculation. Once you have calculated a correlation, you need to evaluate the probability that the resulting r value might represent a spurious result rather than a true correlation. To determine if an r value is significant, you usually consult a correlation table for the Pearson r and these are generally included in most introductory statistics textbooks (e.g., Coladarci et al., 2008). To use a correlation table you need to know the number of participants in a study and a related concept referred to as *degrees of freedom.*[1] The degrees of freedom for a statistic relate to the number of participants but reflect the number of data points that are free to vary or " . . . the number of independent pieces of information a sample of observations can provide" (Coladarci et al., 2008, p. 267). Degrees of freedom for a statistic are always the number of participants minus some number, and for a Pearson r correlation statistic, the degrees of freedom are the number of pairs minus two.

Let's consider the examples in Figure 9–2 and Figure 9–3. The figures illustrate two different associations; however, both hypothetical studies included 25 participants. The measures plotted along the vertical and horizontal axes might be two different ways to measure some aspect of speech, language, or hearing. The researchers selected a random sample of 25 participants and administered both measures to each person. In these examples, the samples included 25 participants; thus, the degrees of freedom for evaluating the significance of the correlation and probability of error would be 23 (25 − 2 or the number of participants/paired scores minus 2). When the researchers consulted a statistical table for the Pearson r, they found that the critical value of r was 0.396 with 23 degrees of freedom and a probability of 0.05. If the computed value of r is greater than or equal to the critical value, 0.396 in our example, the correlation would be significant. If the computed value of r is less than the critical value in the table, the probability of error would be greater than 0.05 and the correlation would be nonsignificant. Therefore, the correlation associated with Figure 9–2 was significant at the 0.05 level, but the one associated with Figure 9–3 was not. Guidelines in the publication manual of the American Psychological Association (APA, 2001) suggest including the statistical symbol, degrees of freedom, computed value, and probability when reporting statistics. The results in Figure 9–2 would be reported as $r(23) = −0.93$, $p < 0.05$, and the results in Figure 9–3 would be reported as $r(23) = 0.25$, $p > 0.05$.

Sample size and degrees of freedom have a strong influence on the likelihood that a computed correlation would be significant. Even a weak correlation could be significant in a statistical sense if the sample size is large enough. For example, if our researchers had a larger sample of 102 participants and 100 degrees of freedom, the critical value for r would be only 0.195 at the 0.05 level. On the other hand, if they had a small sample, perhaps 12 participants and 10 degrees of freedom, the critical value for r would be 0.576. In research, obtaining a result that is statistically significant is not the same as obtaining an important result. If a weak correlation (e.g., $r = 0.25$) is significant, it means that the probability that it occurred because of spurious, random factors is low. However, it does not mean this correlation would be particularly useful to a researcher who wanted to show that two tests measured a skill in highly similar ways.

---

[1]The abbreviation for degrees of freedom is *df* (APA, 2001).

When conducting a significance test, researchers need to keep in mind one caution. The probability of error associated with a level of significance, such as 0.05, usually is for a single test of significance. If a research team conducted a study and computed the correlations among several measures, they need to be cautious about the probability of a type I error. Although the significance level for an individual correlation might be set at 0.05, the probability of a type I error for the entire study could be much higher. The example in Table 9-1 shows a problem with computing several correlation coefficients and making multiple comparisons. In this example, the researcher obtained scores from 5 different measures and wished to determine if these scores were intercorrelated. In this example study the researchers calculated 10 correlation coefficients and tested each for significance at the 0.05 level. The researcher found a single correlation (0.48) with a probability of less than 0.05. How-

ever, a careful researcher would ask if the probability of error was still 0.05 after running 10 different statistical tests, and the answer to that question would be "no." The actual probability of error is much higher and is based on the number of individual correlations. For the example in Table 9-1, you could determine the actual error rate by using the following formula: $p = 1 - (1 - 0.05)^{10}$ (Ottenbacher, 1986). In this formula, the value of $(1 - 0.05)$ is 0.95 and when 0.95 is multiplied by itself 10 times, the resulting value is 0.60. Thus, the actual probability of error in a series of 10 separate correlation computations is $1 - 0.60$ or 0.40 (Jacobs, 1976). This is a 40 in 100 chance of a type I error as compared to the 5 in 100 chance of error that most statistical textbooks recommend. When calculating multiple correlation coefficients, one recommendation is to adopt a more conservative error rate such as 0.01. Researchers should also be highly suspicious of their findings when only one correlation coefficient

Table 9–1. Illustration of a table with several correlation coefficients and the possibility of an inflated error rate

	Speech Discrimination	Phonological Awareness	Consonant Composite	Digit Span
Speech Discrimination				
Phonological Awareness	0.48*			
Consonant Composite	0.36	0.40		
Digit Span	0.22	0.10	0.35	
Picture Vocabulary	0.30	0.30	0.20	0.15

$N = 20$, *$p < 0.05$

in a large table meets the test of significance (i.e., is significant at the 0.05 level).

Another caution in interpreting a significant correlation coefficient is to consider whether a tested relationship makes logical sense. Sometimes you can obtain a significant correlation between two variables that are not directly related. Rather, the two variables both relate to a third variable you did not measure. Consider the hypothetical example of a researcher who measured height in inches and also gave the same children a language test that yielded an age equivalent score. The researcher might obtain a significant correlation between height in inches and language age, but logically these two variables should not be directly related. Children who are relatively tall can have language delays and children who are relatively shorter can be quite expressive. However, if the sample included children across a wide age range, such as from ages 3 to 7, then one would expect to see both growth in height and language age with increases in chronological age. The two variables would appear to be correlated because both height and language age correlated to a third variable, chronological age, that was not evaluated.

Coefficient of Determination

The coefficient of determination is a measure that is closely related to the Pearson r. Its symbol is r^2 (Coladarci et al., 2008; Pyrczak, 2006). Calculation of the coefficient of determination is straightforward; you simply square the Pearson r. Some examples are listed below:

Pearson r	r^2
0.20	0.04
0.50	0.25
0.80	0.64

The coefficient of determination provides information that is helpful in interpreting the magnitude or importance of a correlation. By multiplying a coefficient of determination by 100, a researcher obtains a percentage that reflects the degree of association between two variables. Literally, an r^2 tells you what percentage of variation in one measure can be accounted for by variation in the other measure (Pyrczak, 2006). Consider the correlation depicted in Figure 9-1. If you knew a participant's score on Test 1, you could guess the score on Test 2 and come very close. An r of 0.98 corresponds to an r^2 of 0.96 and knowing one of the scores lets you account for 96% of the variation in the other score. On the other hand, the correlation depicted in Figure 9-3 was weak. An r of 0.25 would only let you account for 6% of the variation in the other measure.

Spearman Rank-Order Correlation

If the level of measurement is ordinal, researchers often use the *Spearman rank-order correlation* coefficient (rho) rather than a Pearson r. The Spearman correlation coefficient is a nonparametric statistic and also might be useful when your data do not meet the assumptions associated with use of the Pearson r. For example, researchers might prefer the Spearman rho if the data have a substantial positive or negative skew. Calculation of a Spearman rho involves comparing two sets of rank-ordered measures (Coladarci et al., 2008; Gibbons & Chakraborti, 2003). The range of values for a Spearman rho is similar to a Pearson r, from 0.0 to ±1.0. The closer the value is to ±1.0, the stronger the correlation; and the closer the value is to 0.0, the weaker the correlation. A value of −1.0 indicates a perfect negative relationship, a +1.0 indicates a perfect positive relationship, and a zero indicates no relationship.

The example in Table 9–2 illustrates two sets of rank-ordered scores and the procedures for calculating a Spearman rho. To compute rho you determine the difference in ranks, square the difference to remove negative values, and then sum the squared ranks. This information is entered into the formula as shown in Table 9–2. Most commercially available statistical applications include a function for computing a Spearman correlation coefficient, but this function might not be available in a basic spreadsheet program. To determine if the statistical value is significant at an appropriate error rate such as 0.05, you look up the critical value in a statistical table as you would for the Pearson r.

Chi Square and Contingency Coefficient

Researchers also have tools for investigating associations among sets of observations when their level of measurement is nominal. One procedure for investigating the degree of association between two categorical variables is a chi square analysis and contingency table (Coladarci et al., 2008; Gibbons & Chakraborti, 2003). The hypothetical example in Table 9–3 illustrates a 2 by 3 contingency table with two variables: area of specialization in communication sciences and disorders and primary factor in employment decisions. The specialization variable has 2 levels and the employment factors variable has 3 levels. The numbers in the table are frequencies and represent the number of persons in a particular category

Table 9–2. Example of using rank-ordered scores in the calculation of a Spearman rank-order correlation coefficient

Participant Identifier	Participant Ranks on Measure 1	Participant Ranks on Measure 2	Difference in Ranks	Difference Squared
A	10	9	1	1
B	2	1	1	1
C	1	2	−1	1
D	6	7	−1	1
E	3	8	−5	25
F	9	10	−1	1
G	7	5	2	4
H	8	4	4	16
I	4	3	1	1
J	5	6	−1	1

Sum of squared differences = 52

Rho = 0.685

Formula for calculating rho is $1 - (6 * 52/(10 * (10^2 - 1))$

Table 9–3. Example of a 3 by 3 contingency table and chi square computation

	Most Important Factor in Employment Decisions			Row Subtotal
	Annual Salary	Work Setting	Other	
Audiologists	80 (Observed) 100 (Expected)	80 60 (Expected)	40 40 (Expected)	200
Speech-Language Pathologists	120 100 (Expected)	40 60 (Expected)	40 40 (Expected)	200
Column Subtotal	200	120	80	Total = 400

Note: The numbers in this table are entirely hypothetical.

Chi square = $((80 - 100)^2 \div 100) + ((80 - 60)^2 \div 60) + ((40 - 40)^2 \div 40) + ((120 - 100)^2 \div 100) + ((40 - 60)^2 \div 60) + ((40 - 40^2) \div 40)$

Chi square = $4 + 6.67 + 0 + 4 + 6.67 + 0$

Chi square = 21.33

Contingency coefficient = square root of $(21.33/400 + 21.33)$ or .225

(e.g., audiologists, speech-language pathologists) who chose each reason for making an employment decision. The logic underlying a chi square is that an association between the two variables would appear as a difference in the observed frequency compared to the *expected* frequency. The expected frequency is similar to a null hypothesis and represents the situation that would occur if the two variables had no association. In our example, the number of audiologists and speech-language pathologists is equal so the expected frequencies reflect equal distribution of the professions under each decision factor. The actual computation uses the value of the following for each cell: (Observed – Expected)^2 ÷ Expected. As with other statistical values, you determine if the probability of error is greater than 0.05 by consulting a chi square table. The degrees of freedom for a chi square are based on the number of rows and columns [(rows – 1) * (columns – 1)]. For the example in Table 9–3 the degrees of freedom would be (2 – 1) * (3 – 1) or 2. Contingency tables with 2 rows and 2 columns are also common, but the table could have different numbers of rows and columns (e.g., 3 by 3, 4 by 3).

Sometimes researchers need to estimate the magnitude of the association between two categorical variables. One way to make such an estimate is to compute a *contingency coefficient* (abbreviated as C) (Pyrczak, 2006). Because contingency coefficients are computed from a chi square, you complete the chi square analysis first and then compute a contingency coefficient from the chi square, wherein C is equal to the square root of (chi square/(N + chi square)). This value is shown in Table 9–3 along with the chi square computation. Contingency coefficients may range from 0 to 1.0 but are distributed differently depending on the size of the contingency table. Thus, 0 to 1.0 reflects the maximum range, and the actual upper limit could be less. For this reason, contingency coefficients cannot be compared directly unless they are yielded by tables of the same size (Pyrczak, 2006). Due to the computation procedures, contingency coefficients are always positive and do not convey information about the direction of a relationship.

Simple Regression and Multiple Regression

Sometimes researchers want to investigate the predictive value of an association. In these instances, they might conduct a regression analysis rather than a correlation analysis. A simple regression with two variables is similar to a correlation, except that one variable is the independent or predictor variable and the other is the dependent variable. A regression analysis allows you to predict or estimate the value of a dependent variable if you know the value of the independent variable. One thing researchers might do is generate a regression line to show where predicted scores would fall. This possibility is illustrated in Figure 9–4. These are the same data portrayed in Figure 9–1, but in this case we added a regression line to the display and designated the variable along the X-axis as the independent variable (predictor) and the variable along the Y-axis as the dependent variable (predicted). The slope of the line represents the amount of change in Y that corresponds to a change of one unit in X. The regression line is the line of "best fit" or the line about which the scores would deviate the least.

In the case of a simple regression with two variables, the regression statistic (r^2) and the Pearson r relate to one another in a direct way. The regression statistic is the square of the Pearson r. You might recall this value from our discussion of the coefficient of determination. However, in the case of a regression, you might think of the r^2 as reflecting the extent to which changes in the Y variable are predictable if you know the person's score on the X variable. One common use of regression analysis is to determine the value of the independent (X) variable for predicting future performance on the dependent (Y) variable. An example of this would be research in the area of reading where researchers have investigated the predictive value of various measures of phonemic awareness to determine if they

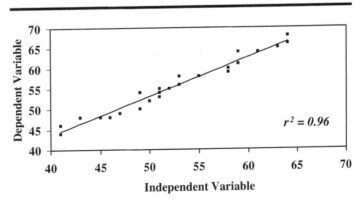

Figure 9–4. An illustration of a simple regression model with one dependent variable and one independent variable and a linear regression line representing the predicted relationship between the two variables.

would provide early identification of children who would be at risk for reading problems in the future. In this example, measures of phonemic awareness would be the independent variables and measures of reading skills would be the dependent variables.

Sometimes questions about the relationships among variables are too complex to analyze with a simple regression model. For example, a researcher might be interested in investigating the simultaneous prediction value of two or more independent variables; or perhaps a researcher discovered that the independent and dependent variables in a study are related in a nonlinear manner. Simple regression works well for investigating the prediction relationship between two variables whose relationship roughly approximates a straight line, but for the more complex examples, a researcher might consider using a *multiple regression* analysis and/or a *nonlinear regression* analysis (Velleman, 1997).

Multiple regression techniques allow you to determine the strongest combination of variables for predicting outcomes on a dependent variable. Often with regression analysis researchers are interested in predicting a future outcome. Our simple regression example involved predicting future reading skills from a measure of phonemic awareness. Another example might be predicting future speech sound production abilities of preschool children with hearing impairment. Perhaps researchers have developed a new way to test speech discrimination abilities of young children at ages 3 and 4. They also know the children's average pure-tone thresholds. The researchers want to determine if one or both of these measures would enable them to accurately predict speech production abilities at age 6, as measured by the percentage of intelligible words in conversational speech. Such a study would require a longitudinal research

design because the researchers need to measure the *independent* variables at ages 3 and 4, and then reassess the children at age 6 to determine their speech intelligibility. Once they have collected these measures, the researchers can complete a multiple regression analysis with speech intelligibility as the dependent variable and speech discrimination and average pure-tone threshold as independent variables. The results of the regression analysis will provide information to determine the strength of the predictive relationship, expressed as an r^2, the probability of error associated with the analysis, and the extent to which each of the independent variables made a significant contribution to the prediction. The computation and interpretation for a multiple regression analysis are complex and those who might need to use such an analysis need to consult more advanced data analysis textbooks (e.g., Rosenthal & Rosnow, 2008; StatSoft, Inc., 2007; Woods, Fletcher, & Hughes, 1986).

One final consideration in designing a regression analysis is whether or not the relationships among the dependent and independent variables are linear. Some variables might actually have a highly predictable relationship, but because the relationship is curvilinear rather than linear, a simple regression on the variables would yield disappointing findings. Figure 9–5 illustrates one example of a curvilinear relationship. This type of curve sometimes is called an *inverted U* shape, but more formally it is a quadratic relationship (Velleman, 1997). If you completed a simple regression and obtained an r^2 for these two variables, the value would be very low, $r^2 = 0.006$. This would mean that only 0.6% of the variability in the dependent variable could be accounted for by its relationship with the independent or predictor variable. However, the two variables are actually more closely

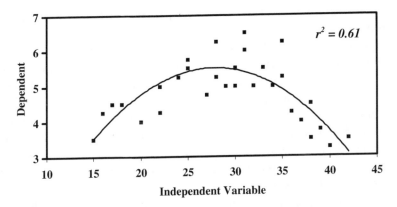

Figure 9–5. An illustration of a nonlinear relationship with one dependent variable and one independent variable and a line of best fit representing the curvilinear relationship.

related than that. The problem is that both low scores and high scores on the independent variable are associated with low scores on the dependent variable, whereas mid-range scores on the independent variable are associated with high scores on the dependent variable. If the researcher used an appropriate type of nonlinear regression to analyze this relationship, the resulting r^2 would be much larger, $r^2 = 0.61$. This means that the relationship between the independent and dependent variables, when treated as a nonlinear relationship, accounted for 61% of the variability. This example illustrates two important points about data analysis. First, examining a graphic display of your data is helpful for determining how to approach the analysis. This is one way to determine important characteristics such as the linearity of relationships and the shapes of distributions. Second, choosing an appropriate analysis procedure has a definite impact on the accuracy of your findings. An inappropriate analysis might mask a relationship that actually exists in the data.

Thus far our discussion of data analysis has focused on procedures for investigating associations among variables. In this type of study, researchers study a single group of participants and obtain two or more measures from each participant. Studies that employ correlation and regression analyses are usually nonexperimental designs in which the researchers examine preexisting relationships among variables. The next section focuses on data analysis procedures for examining differences between groups. Although difference tests are useful for analyzing group differences in nonexperimental designs (Woods et al., 1986), one of their main uses is in analyzing results from randomized experimental designs.

Testing for Differences between Two Samples

Many statistical tests are available for analyzing differences between groups. In deciding which test is most appropriate, you need to consider how many groups you are going to compare, as well as what kind of differences you are analyzing. Additionally, some statistical tests are best for interval and ratio level measurements, observations that fit certain assumptions about the distribution of data around the mean, and larger sample sizes. These are called parametric statistics (StatSoft, 2007). Other statistical tests, called nonparametric statistics, are best for ordinal level measurements, situations where you are uncertain about the distribution of data, and smaller sample sizes (Gibbons & Chakraborti, 2003). Thus, researchers also need to consider whether a parametric or nonparametric statistic would be a better choice for analyzing their data.

Independent and Paired *t*-Tests

The *t*-test is the most common procedure used for analyzing the difference between two sets of data when you have interval or ratio level measures. A *t*-test specifically tests the difference between means to determine if two groups are significantly different. Figure 9–6 and Figure 9–7 illustrate the types of group differences that could be analyzed with a *t*-test. Each figure contains a frequency polygon for two different groups. In each instance the group means are 10 points apart, as shown by the arrows, and in each

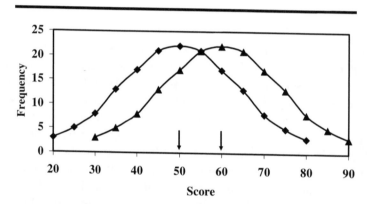

Figure 9–6. A frequency polygon illustrating the difference between means for two groups with relatively greater variability among scores.

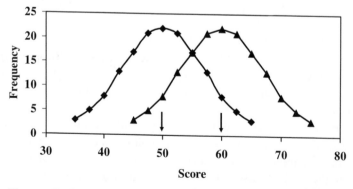

Figure 9–7. A frequency polygon illustrating the difference between means for two groups with relatively less variability among scores.

instance the groups partially overlap. However, the two groups represented in Figure 9-6 overlap more than the two groups in Figure 9-7. This greater overlap occurs because the scores in Figure 9-6 are more widely dispersed around the mean. Whenever researchers analyze data with a t-test, they are trying to determine if an observed difference between groups means is a true difference. A significant result means that the observed difference is most likely a real difference with a low probability of error (e.g., less than 0.05 or less than 0.01).

Three factors influence whether or not you will find a significant difference when analyzing data with a t-test (Pyrczak, 2006). One of these factors is the magnitude of the difference between means. All other factors being equal, the larger the difference between means, the more likely the t-test analysis will come out significant. A second factor that influences the likelihood of obtaining a significant outcome is the amount of variability in your data. The less variable the scores, as measured by variance and standard deviation, the more likely a difference between means will come out significant. Figure 9-6 and Figure 9-7 both illustrate situations in which the groups differ by 10 points. However, the groups illustrated in Figure 9-6 have greater variance than the groups in Figure 9-7. When scores are more widely dispersed around the mean, you need a larger mean difference to obtain significance. Sample size is a final factor that influences whether or not a statistical analysis will yield a significant result. The larger the sample size, the more likely the outcome of an analysis will be significant. Recall from the chapter on sampling that a larger random sample is more likely to represent the population well than a smaller random sample.

The data in Table 9-4 illustrate how sample size and variability influence probability of error and significance testing. The first four columns present scores randomly selected from distributions similar to the ones depicted in Figure 9-6. Columns 1 and 2 are relatively larger samples ($n = 25$), whereas columns 3 and 4 are relatively smaller samples. The group means differ by approximately 10 points and the data in columns 1 through 4 are relatively more variable with standard deviations of 10.8 and above. The last four columns present scores randomly selected from distributions similar to the ones depicted in Figure 9-7. Again, the group means differ by approximately 10 points; however, the data in columns 5 through 8 are less variable as reflected by the smaller standard deviations. Although computing a t-test by hand is possible, it is safer to use a spreadsheet statistical function or dedicated statistical software for the task. The results reported in Table 9-4 are from a dedicated statistical software package, DataDesk (2003).

When using t-tests you need to consider whether the two samples being compared are related or independent. Related samples are either two measures on the same participants, such as measures at two different times, or measures from samples of matched participants. Sometimes researchers create participant pairs by matching them on some pretest measure. After the matching the researchers randomly assign the participants to one of two treatment groups. With either two measures on the same participants or matched participants, the appropriate t-test is a *paired t-test*. With independent samples, the appropriate t-test is an *independent t-test*. One way this choice affects your analysis is when you determine degrees of freedom. The degrees of freedom for a paired t-test are the number of pairs minus one ($n - 1$). If you had 25 matched participants, the degrees of freedom for your analysis would be 24. For an independent t-test you have two options for determining degrees of freedom. The

Table 9–4. Example of computation of t-tests for more and less variable groups with different sample sizes

	More Variable				Less Variable			
	$n = 25$		$n = 10$		$n = 25$		$n = 10$	
	1st	*2nd*	*3rd*	*4th*	*5th*	*6th*	*7th*	*8th*
	57	70	57	70	55	67	55	67
	33	49	33	49	55	65	55	65
	47	49	47	49	39	50	39	50
	40	50	40	50	40	51	40	51
	40	44	40	44	57	67	57	67
	51	58	51	58	60	70	60	70
	52	69	52	69	52	61	52	61
	38	51	38	51	45	54	45	54
	57	67	57	67	43	53	43	53
	73	73	73	73	59	69	59	69
	33	48			40	48		
	67	75			49	61		
	47	52			45	53		
	49	64			49	59		
	60	72			56	65		
	43	53			52	64		
	29	31			50	59		
	64	72			51	62		
	61	73			44	56		
	62	75			45	55		
	69	82			54	65		
	39	52			57	67		
	55	72			49	60		
	50	50			59	69		
	27	41			40	49		
$M =$	49.6	59.6	48.7	57.9	49.8	60.0	50.5	60.8
$SD =$	12.9	13.4	11.8	10.8	6.7	6.9	7.9	8.0

most common when you have equal numbers of participants in each group is called the *pooled variance* t-test. You add the number of participants in each group and subtract 2 ($n_1 + n_2 - 2$). If you had 25 participants in each group the degrees of freedom would be 25 + 25 - 2 or 48. When you have two independent samples, and the variances of the two groups are different, using the pooled variance t-test is inappropriate. Determining the degrees of freedom for groups with different variances is beyond the scope of our discussion. You might consult other sources if confronted with this situation (Velleman, 1997).

Let's return to the data in Table 9-4. These data represent independent samples, so we are going to analyze the mean differences using an independent t-test. First, we are going to report the results for the larger samples ($n = 25$). Pyrczak (2006) recommends always reporting the values of your means and standard deviations before reporting the results of a t-test, so this information is included in Table 9-4. The results from the analysis of the more variable groups revealed a significant difference between the first and second groups, $t (48) = -2.69$, $p < 0.01$. Repeating the analysis for the data in columns 5 and 6 revealed a significant difference between the fifth and sixth groups as well, $t (48) = -5.33, p < 0.0001$.[2] Thus, with samples of 25 participants the differences between groups were significant for both the more variable and less variable samples.

Let's repeat our analyses with the smaller samples, starting with the more variable groups in columns 3 and 4. In this case our degrees of freedom will be 10 + 10 − 2 or 18. The results from this analysis revealed the mean difference between the third and fourth groups was not significant at the 0.05 level, $t (18) = -1.82, p = 0.09$. Finally, let's complete our example by analyzing the data in columns 7 and 8. The results from the analysis of the less variable groups revealed a significant difference between the seventh and eighth groups, $t (18) = -2.86, p = 0.01$. The t-test results reported here follow the guidelines in the APA (2001) publication manual by including the statistical symbol, degrees of freedom, statistical value, and probability.

Sometimes researchers want to investigate the differences between two groups but find that using a t-test would be inappropriate. One reason could be that the level of measurement was ordinal rather than interval or ratio. Otherwise, the researchers might be concerned that their data do not meet the assumptions associated with a parametric test such as a t-test. Perhaps their sample sizes are quite small, or they are uncertain how their measures distribute about the mean. For example, they might have noted an obvious positive or negative skew in a plot of the scores. In these situations, alternative, nonparametric procedures such as the Mann-Whitney U test, sign test, or the Wilcoxon signed-ranks test might be better choices for analyzing the data.

In Chapter 6 we covered different experimental designs. Each of those designs would correspond to one of the data analysis procedures we are covering in this chapter. An independent t-test might be used to analyze data from a randomized, posttest-only design. An independent t-test also might be appropriate for analyzing data from a nonexperimental design, such as when researchers compare random samples from two populations with preexisting differences. In the field of communication sciences and disorders, studies often focus on comparing persons with a communication disorder and those with typical communication skills. If only two groups are being compared, an independent t-test would be one way to analyze the data.

---

[2]Many dedicated statistical software packages report the actual probability of error, and the p values reported by DataDesk® are included here.

Mann-Whitney *U*

The Mann-Whitney *U* test is a nonparametric test that is appropriate for testing the difference between two independent groups (Gibbons & Chakraborti, 2003). This test can be used with ordinal, ranked scores or you can convert a set of measures to ranks. An example of the setup and computation of a Mann-Whitney *U* is shown in Table 9–5. In this hypothetical study, some graduate students conducted a small study to test the effectiveness of a new treatment procedure. They were able to randomly assign their participants to groups, but the sample sizes were small and the groups had different numbers of participants. The students were advised by a statistical consultant at their university to use a Mann-Whitney *U* test to analyze their data. Computing this statistic is relatively easy, as shown in Table 9–5. However, the students used a statistics software program to complete their analysis. In calculation of a Mann-Whitney *U*, the scores of the two groups are ranked as if they were from a single group, and then the ranks for the smaller group are summed (e.g., R_1 in the table). If the two groups are different, the highest ranks should cluster in one group, whereas the lowest ranks should cluster in the other group. The sum of the ranks is entered into a special formula for computation of the *U* statistic (Popham & Sirotnik, 1973, p. 297), as shown in Table 9–5. In our example study, the students found that the higher ranking scores tended to occur in the experimental group and that this difference was significant, $U = 3$, $p = 0.0003$. The statistical analysis software reported the *p* value as well as the value of the *U* statistic. If the students had looked up the value in a statistical table, they would have used the number of participants in each of the two groups to determine the critical value of *U*. For $n_1 = 8$ and $n_2 = 10$, the critical value for *U* at the 0.05 level was 17. The computed value had to be less than or equal to the value in the table, so the *U* of 3 was significant.

Table 9–5. Example computation of a Mann-Whitney *U* test for examining the difference between two independent samples

Treatment Procedure			
Traditional		Experimental	
Score	Rank	Score	Rank
33	4	47	12
30	2	55	18
45	10	42	8
31	3	48	13
20	1	51	16
34	5	49	14
36	7	50	15
46	11	52	17
44	9		
35	6		
		$R_1 = 113$	

$U = n_1 n_2 + n_1 (n_1 + 1)/2 - R_1$ (Popham & Sirotnik, 1973, p. 297)

$U = 10 * 8 + 8(8 + 1)/2 - 113$

$U = 3$, $p = 0.0003$

Sign Test and Wilcoxon Matched-Pairs Signed-Ranks Test

If your scores are from related samples, such as two scores from the same participants, the sign test and the Wilcoxon matched-pairs signed-rank test are useful statistical tests. Like the Mann-Whitney *U* test, these two procedures would be appropriate for ordinal level measures or in situations where the distribution of scores around the mean is irregular (Gibbons & Chakraborti, 2003). The sign test and the Wilcoxon test are nonparametric alternatives to a paired t-test. The sign test is the simplest to compute but only reflects the direction of a difference and not the magnitude of the difference. Consider the situation depicted in Table 9–6. In this example, participants listened to two computer-generated voices and chose the one they preferred. The + or − signs represent the direction of these differences. As long as you are consistent in making the comparisons, the value will be the same. For example, if A was designated as the − and B as the +, the value of x would be the same because you still would count the less frequent sign. With 10 participants and an x of 1, the probability would be 0.011, indi-

cating that the subjects preferred voice A over voice B significantly more often.

The Wilcoxon matched-pairs signed-rank test uses rank-ordered level measurement in its computation. An example of the use of this test is shown in Table 9–7. In this example, the researchers matched their participants on their pretest scores and then randomly assigned one participant from each pair to the computer activity and one to the paper and pencil activity. They found that scores were higher with the computer activity for 8 out of 10 participants. To compute the Wilcoxon matched-pairs signed-rank test (T) statistic, you determine the difference between the scores of the matched pairs, rank those differences with their sign, and then determine the sign (+/−) that occurred less frequently. The T statistic is the sum of the ranks with the less frequently occurring sign, $T = 3$ in our example. For some sample sizes you simply look up the probability associated with T in a table. For example, Gibbons and Chakraborti (2003) include a table for sample sizes up to 15. For larger samples the computation is complex, and the safest approach would be to complete the calculation using a statistics software program.

Table 9–6. Example computation of a sign test for examining the difference between two related samples

Participant	Preferred Voice	Sign
1	A	+
2	A	+
3	A	+
4	A	+
5	B	−
6	A	+
7	A	+
8	A	+
9	A	+
10	A	+

$x = 1^*$ (Count the number of the less frequent sign to obtain x.)

$^*p = 0.011$

Testing for Differences among Three or More Samples

If the design of a study involves three or more groups, usually the technique for data analysis will be an *analysis of variance* (ANOVA). In one sense the analysis of variance is an extension of the t-test, because the outcome is affected by the same factors: mean differences among the groups, amount of variability within and across the groups, and sample size. Although researchers could use an ANOVA to analyze differences

Table 9–7. Example computation of the Wilcoxon matched-pairs signed-rank test for examining the difference between two related samples

| Type of Activity | | | | |
Computer	Paper and Pencil	Difference	Rank of Difference	Less Frequent Sign
51	41	10	8	
65	61	4	4	
40	42	−2	−2	2
60	51	9	7	
38	39	−1	−1	1
63	51	12	10	
65	58	7	5	
57	54	3	3	
58	50	8	6	
50	39	11	9	

Sum the ranks of the less frequent sign, ignoring the sign: $T = 3^*$.

$^*p = 0.005$

Significance of value obtained from Gibbons & Chakraborti (2003, p. 578)

between two groups, this is seldom the practice. Usually ANOVA analyses are reserved for designs with several groups or designs with more than one independent variable.

One of the simplest designs for a *one-way ANOVA* is illustrated in Figure 9–8. This shows three different frequency polygons, each representing a different group. The distributions are roughly normal with scores spreading in a symmetrical way around the group means. An ANOVA computation involves a comparison of different sources of variance in the data. In the example in Figure 9–8, one source of variance is the dispersion of scores around the individual group means. A second source of variance is the overall dispersion of scores across all three groups. If the groups are different, then the overall spread of scores will

be much larger than the spread of scores within the individual groups (StatSoft, 2007). When you examine Figure 9–8, the three groups stand out and are easy to identify. A different situation occurs in Figure 9–9. The three groups overlap to a great extent and are not clearly separated. The overall variance across all three groups and the variance for each individual group are similar, and it is more difficult to identify the three separate groups. A researcher conducting an ANOVA on data similar to that shown in Figure 9–8 would be much more likely to identify a significant difference among the groups than a researcher with data similar to that shown in Figure 9–9.

Analyzing data using analysis of variance is appropriate if you have interval or ratio level measures. The statistic associated

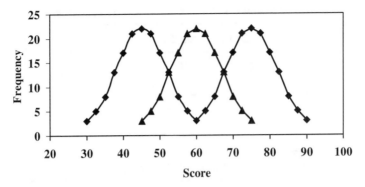

Figure 9–8. A frequency polygon illustrating differences among three groups associated with mean differences and amount of variability.

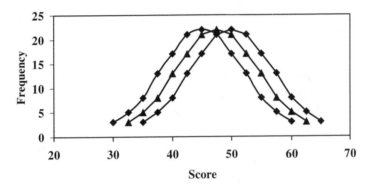

Figure 9–9. A frequency polygon illustrating three groups with relatively greater overlap associated with lesser mean differences relative to variability.

with an ANOVA is an *F* test (Pyrczak, 2006). This statistic is sometimes called an *F* ratio because its computation takes into account the variance associated with differences among groups in relation to the error variance. Like *t*-tests, different ANOVA models are available for analyzing independent groups versus repeated measures from the same participants.

Next, let's review an example of a one-way ANOVA with a single between-groups independent variable. The design in this example is an extension of the randomiz-

ed posttest-only design we analyzed with a *t*-test. The difference is that we now have three independent groups: an experimental treatment group, a traditional treatment group, and a no-treatment control group. The means and standard deviations for each group, along with the results from a one-way ANOVA, are shown in Table 9-8. The computational procedures for an ANOVA are complex, so the results in Table 9-8 are from a statistical software package (Data-Desk, 2003). From the standpoint of the researchers, the most important number in

Table 9–8. Example of a one-way analysis of variance (ANOVA) with three groups

Descriptive Statistics			
	M	**SD**	**n**
Experimental Treatment	46.5	5.53	12
Traditional Treatment	40.1	5.50	12
No Treatment Control	39.8	5.51	12

Analysis of Variance					
Source	**df**	**Sums of Squares**	**Mean Square**	**F-Ratio**	**Probability**
Groups	2	296.72	148.36	4.88	0.014
Error	33	1003.17	30.40		
Total	35	1299.89			

df = degrees of freedom.

the ANOVA table is the probability. With a p of 0.014 they know that probability of error in concluding that there is a difference among the three groups is low, less than 5 in 100. For the purposes of reporting their results, the researchers also would want to know the value of the F ratio and the degrees of freedom for the Groups and Error sources. Note that the total degrees of freedom are the number of participants minus one. The degrees of freedom for Groups are the number of groups minus one. What is left over represents the error degrees of freedom (e.g., $36 - 1 - 2 = 33$). When reporting the results of the analysis in Table 9–8, you would first report the means and standard deviations for each group (Pyrczak, 2006), and then the following: $F (2, 33) = 4.88, p = 0.014$. This format follows the APA (2001) guidelines.

If you obtain a significant result after conducting an ANOVA, you know that one or more of the group differences were significant. However, you do not know exactly which group differences were the significant ones. Examining descriptive statistics, such as the group means and standard deviations,

generally is not sufficient for identifying the specific differences. Rather, researchers follow up a significant ANOVA result with an additional *post hoc* statistical test (i.e., one conducted after the initial analysis). Several different procedures are available specifically for post hoc analysis and making multiple comparisons among means. Some examples include the Bonferroni correction, the Scheffé test, and Tukey's Honest Significant Difference (HSD) test (Coladarci et al., 2008; Velleman, 1997). Examples that follow in a later section of this chapter include use of the Scheffé post hoc test.

A different version of the ANOVA test, a repeated measures ANOVA, is available for situations in which researchers obtained several measures from the same participants. Sometimes these kinds of designs involve participants being observed under three or more experimental conditions. Another application of this kind of design is to obtain repeated measures over time to document growth and/or change with treatment. In the chapter on experimental research design, we noted that a one-group pretest-posttest design was a weak, preexperimental design. One of the major problems with this design is that participants could change over time due to maturation and/or recovery. Such changes would confound any treatment effects you hoped to observe. Trochim & Donnelly (2007) noted that adding a second pretest before initiating treatment was a way to at least partially address this issue. Our example of a one-way repeated measures ANOVA, shown in Table 9–9, is an analysis of this type of design. The researchers recruited 12 participants for an exploratory treatment study. Because they were not able to use random assignment to treatment and control groups, they decided to add a second pretest to their design. As with the example in Table 9–8, these data were analyzed using a statistics software package (DataDesk, 2003). The means and standard deviations for each time, along with the results from a one-way repeated measures ANOVA, are included. The results of the analysis revealed a significant difference in the participants'

performance over time, $F(2, 22) = 37.73$, $p \leq 0.0001$. In this example, the researchers would want to use a post hoc test to verify that the participants did not make a significant change between Pretest 1 and Pretest 2 and that the only difference occurred on the posttest after treatment.

You might examine the ANOVA tables in Table 9–8 and Table 9–9 and identify some of the similarities and differences between the one-way ANOVA for independent groups and the repeated measures ANOVA. Both analyses include similar information: degrees of freedom, sum of squares, mean square, F-ratio, and probability. The variance in the scores is divided among several sources. However, in the case of the repeated measures analysis of variance, an additional source associated with participants was added. This reduced the number of degrees of freedom associated with the error source (i.e., total of $35 - 11 - 2$ for error degrees of freedom). The F-ratio is still the mean square for times divided by the mean square for error.

Table 9–9. Example of a one-way repeated measures analysis of variance (ANOVA) with measures from the same participants at three different times

Descriptive Statistics			
	M	**SD**	**n**
Pretest 1	46.0	5.89	12
Pretest 2	45.3	5.79	12
Posttest	52.2	5.81	12

Analysis of Variance					
Source	**df**	**Sums of Squares**	**Mean Square**	**F-Ratio**	**Probability**
Participants	11	1023.00	93.00	20.60	≤ 0.0001
Times	2	340.67	170.33	37.73	≤ 0.0001
Error	22	99.33	4.52		
Total	35	1463.00			

df = degrees of freedom.

If your level of measurement is ordinal or you have concerns that your data do not meet the assumptions associated with an ANOVA, you might consider one of the nonparametric alternatives to the one-way ANOVA. Nonparametric tests are available to analyze both related and unrelated samples. *Friedman's two-way analysis of variance* is appropriate if you have repeated measures from the same participants or related samples due to matching. Although this test is called a two-way analysis of variance, it is an alternative to a one-way repeated measures ANOVA. A second nonparametric test, the *Kruskal-Wallis test*, is an equivalent of a one-way ANOVA for independent samples. Gibbons and Chakraborti (2003) provide a detailed discussion of the nature and computation of these nonparametric alternatives.

Statistical Analysis for Factorial Designs

A one-way analysis of variance is useful for studies with one independent variable or factor. Although the example in Table 9–8 had three levels of the independent variable, such an analysis could compare even more groups. However, sometimes researchers want to investigate two or more independent variables in the same study. We learned in Chapter 6 that designs with more than one independent variable are factorial designs. The analyses for these designs are called two-way ANOVAs, three-way ANOVAs, and so forth, depending on the number of factors or independent variables. Theoretically, researchers could design a study with many different independent variables. However, practically you seldom see more than four or five different factors, and even those

designs are relatively rare. The interpretation of multiway ANOVAs is complex and the more variables you add, the more challenging it becomes to explain your findings.

The example in Table 9–10 illustrates a 2 by 2 analysis of variance. This is one of the simplest factorial designs. The notation *2 by 2* means you have two independent variables and each of those variables has two levels. In this example, the independent variables are intensity of treatment and type of treatment. The levels for the intensity variable are two sessions per week and four sessions per week, and the levels for type of treatment are experimental and traditional. The researchers randomly assigned 10 participants to each treatment/intensity combination. Although this study has two independent variables, the design is still a randomized posttest-only design because the researchers only tested their participants one time at the end of treatment.

The ANOVA table is shown at the bottom of Table 9–10, and much of the information is familiar from our discussion of one-way analysis of variance: degrees of freedom, sums of squares, mean square, *F*-ratio, and probability. In the case of this two-way ANOVA, the sources of variance include the two independent variables, intensity and treatment, and an additional source called the intensity-by-treatment (int. by trt.) interaction. Any differences associated with the two independent variables often are called *main effects*, and differences associated with the intensity-by-treatment interaction are called *interaction effects*.

A two-way ANOVA would enable you to determine if there are differences associated with your main effects (the main levels), as well as any interactions between the levels. For the example in Table 9–10, the main effects for intensity of treatment [$F(1, 36) = 10.77$, $p = 0.0023$] and type of treat-

Table 9–10. Example of a two-way analysis of variance (ANOVA) with two independent variables, treatment type and intensity

Descriptive Statistics

	Two sessions/week	Four sessions/week
Experimental	$M = 13.60$ $SD = 4.60$ $n = 10$	$M = 23.20$ $SD = 4.54$ $n = 10$
Traditional	$M = 13.40$ $SD = 4.62$ $n = 10$	$M = 13.30$ $SD = 4.55$ $n = 10$

Analysis of Variance

Source	df	Sums of Squares	Mean Square	F-Ratio	Probability
Intensity	1	225.63	225.63	10.77	0.0023
Treatment	1	255.03	255.03	12.17	0.0013
Int. by Trt.	1	235.23	235.23	11.22	0.0019
Error	36	754.50	20.96		
Total	39	1470.37			

df = degrees of freedom.

ment [$F(1, 36) = 12.17, p = 0.0013$] were significant, as well as the intensity-by-treatment interaction [$F(1, 36) = 11.22, p = 0.0010$]. A significant interaction means that the outcome for one of the independent variables was different depending on the level of the other independent variable. In our example, the outcome for treatment was different depending on the level of intensity. When you have a significant interaction it is good practice to examine this source first rather than focus on the main effects. A beginning step in analyzing an interaction is to plot the individual group or cell means, and a line graph is a useful tool for generating this plot. Figure 9–10 shows the interaction of treatment and intensity. As shown in this graph, the mean for the experimen-

tal treatment was greater than the mean for traditional treatment when the treatment was intense (four times per week) but not when the treatment was less frequent. Researchers also use post hoc tests such as the Scheffé test and Tukey's HSD test to further analyze significant interactions as well. These post hoc tests are designed to tell you which individual group comparisons were significant. The results for the Scheffé test as reported by DataDesk (2003) revealed the following significant differences:

1. Difference between two sessions and four sessions per week for the experiment treatment was 9.60, $p < 0.0001$
2. Difference between traditional treatment with two sessions per week and

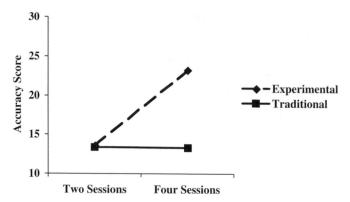

Figure 9–10. A line graph illustrating an interacting between type of treatment and intensity of treatment.

experimental treatment with four sessions per week was 9.80, $p < 0.0001$

3. Difference between traditional treatment and experimental treatment with four sessions per week was 9.90, $p < 0.0001$

Hypothetically, an interaction such as the one illustrated in Figure 9–10 could occur with persons with communication disorders. Perhaps a subgroup did not respond well to traditional treatment, so researchers decided to study an experimental treatment program. The experimental program was not effective either, unless it was presented more intensely. On the other hand, more intense treatment did not improve the effectiveness of the traditional treatment approach.

The final example, shown in Table 9–11, is an analysis of a randomized pretest-posttest design. The analysis procedure for a randomized pretest-posttest design is a *mixed model ANOVA*. The procedure is called a mixed model because it has both a repeated measure factor, the pretest and posttest, and a between group factor, experimental or traditional treatment. In a mixed model ANOVA one source of variance is associated with participants. The other sources are associated with the between group factor (treatments), the repeated measures factors (time of test), the interactions (treatments by time), and the error term. In this analysis of a randomized pretest-posttest design, only the main effect for time of test was significant [F (1,18) = 105.35, $p < 0.0001$]. Examination of the means and standard deviations at the top of the table revealed that both the experimental and traditional treatment groups improved from the pretest to posttest, and the amount of improvement was approximately equal. This type of design and analysis is particularly important in the field of communication sciences and disorders because it often is employed in randomized clinical trials.

Summary

Inferential statistics is a valuable tool for helping researchers determine the likelihood that their observations, based on a small sample, represent the actual situation in a population. Statistical tests provide

Table 9–11. Example of a two-way mixed-model analysis of variance (ANOVA) with one between and one repeated measures variable

	Descriptive Statistics	
	Pretest	**Posttest**
Experimental	$M = 6.80$	$M = 13.70$
	$SD = 2.30$	$SD = 2.31$
	$n = 10$	$n = 10$
Traditional	$M = 6.70$	$M = 13.20$
	$SD = 2.31$	$SD = 2.35$
	$n = 10$	$n = 10$

		Analysis of Variance			
Source	*df*	**Sums of Squares**	**Mean Square**	*F*-Ratio	**Probability**
Participants	18	116.70	6.48	1.52	0.1908
Treatments	1	0.90	0.90	0.14	0.7138
Time	1	448.90	448.90	105.35	≤ 0.0001
Trt. by Time	1	0.40	0.40	0.09	0.7628
Error	18	76.70	4.26		
Total	39	643.60			

df = degrees of freedom.

information about the probability that results reflect the "true" situation in a population or a spurious finding associated with some idiosyncrasy in the sample. Inferential statistics provides information about the probability of error. Thus, if a statistic is significant at the 0.05 level, it means that the probability of error is less than 5 in 100.

Measures of association are statistical tools for investigating the relationship between two or more measures. These measures usually yield information about the strength of a relationship as well as whether it is a direct or inverse relationship. Some example of measures of association are the Pearson product-moment correlation coefficient for interval and ratio level data, the Spearman rank-order correla-

tion coefficient for ordinal level data, and the chi square analysis for nominal data.

Simple regression and multiple regression are ways of analyzing associations among variables for the purpose of making predictions. In a simple regression, one variable is the independent or predictor variable and the other is the dependent variable. The simple regression statistic, an r^2, has a direct relationship to the Pearson r. Other types of regression such as multiple regression and nonlinear regression are useful when researchers want to explore the predictive value of more than one independent variable or to analyze variables that have a curvilinear relationship.

Many statistical tests are designed to test the differences between groups. The *t*-test is one of the most common analysis procedures when the comparison involves two sets of scores. Different versions of the *t*-test are available for independent samples and matched or related samples. When the design of a study involves three or more groups, the most common data analysis procedure is an analysis of variance (ANOVA). A one-way ANOVA is appropriate for analyzing experimental research with one independent variable that has three or more levels, such as a no-treatment control group, a traditional treatment group, and an experimental treatment group. Like a *t*-test, different versions of the one-way ANOVA are available for analyzing independent samples and repeated measures on the same participants. When researchers want to investigate two or more independent variables in the same study, the choice of analysis procedure usually is a multiway analysis of variance. If the study has two independent variables, the analysis is a two-way ANOVA, if the study has three independent variables, the analysis is a three-way ANOVA, and so forth. A special version of a multiway analysis of variance, called a mixed model ANOVA, is particularly important for conducting clinical research. A two-way mixed model ANOVA would have one between group independent variable and one repeated measure variable. This type of analysis is appropriate for randomized pretest-posttest designs. In this kind of design the pretest and posttest are repeated measures and the experimental treatment is the between group variable.

Review Questions

1. What does it mean when a researcher reports that the probability for a statistic was $p < 0.01$?

2. What does it mean when a researcher reports that the probability for a statistic was $p > 0.05$?

3. When the relationship between two variables is perfect and inverse, what is the value of *r*?

4. Is an *r* of −0.90 stronger than an *r* of 0.50? Explain.

5. For a Pearson *r* of 0.50, what is the value of the coefficient of determination? What does this coefficient mean?

6. If you read that the value of a Pearson *r* is 0.45, $p > 0.05$, should you have confidence that this correlation represents the actual situation in the population? Why or why not?

7. If you make an error of rejecting the null hypothesis when it is true, what type of error have you made?

8. Which is the higher level of significance, 0.01 or 0.001?

9. Would you say that the following is *statistically significant* or *not statistically significant*? ($r = 0.40$, $df = 18$, $p > 0.05$)

10. What is the difference between a simple regression and a multiple regression?

11. What difference is tested for significance using a *t*-test?

12. Identify three factors that affect whether or not the results of a *t*-test will be significant.

13. If you are conducting a *t*-test on two scores from the same subjects, or scores from a matched sample, what kind of *t*-test will you use?

14. What nonparametric statistic can be used to test the difference between two groups when you have independent samples?

15. If you have two random samples with 12 subjects in each, how many degrees of freedom do you have for the *t*-test?

16. If you read the following, $t(18) = 1.38$, $p > 0.05$, what conclusion would you make?

17. What are two reasons that you might select a nonparametric alternative to a *t*-test, such as the Wilcoxon signed rank test or the Mann-Whitney U test?

18. You had a sample with six matched pairs of participants. One participant from each pair was randomly assigned to treatment A, and the other to treatment B. The participants' scores are listed below. Show how you would compute the sign test for these data.

Score for Subject Receiving Treatment A	Score for Subject Receiving Treatment B
56	62
50	52
53	49
48	54
57	61
51	59

19. Interpret the parts of the following one-way ANOVA statistic: $F(2,43) = 6.45$, $p < 0.05$.

20. Explain what it means when you have a significant interaction in an ANOVA analysis.

Learning Activities

1. The analysis in Table 9–12 is from a hypothetical study comparing performance of children with communication disorders, their chronological age-matched peers, and their communication age-matched peers. The study had two independent variables: a group variable that was nonexperimental and a method variable that was experimental. The information reported includes descriptive statistics for the three groups of children across the two methods. The inferential data analysis was a two-way analysis of variance (ANOVA) with group and method as the independent variables. First, examine the descriptive statistics. What do you think might have happened in this study? You might consider entering the means in a spreadsheet and generating a bar graph or line graph. Second, examine the ANOVA table. What information in this table is important? Write out the statistical results in the style recommended by the American Psychological Association (2001). Would you need to complete post hoc testing with these results? Explain.

Table 9–12. Hypothetical study comparing performance of children with communication disorders (CD), their chronological age-matched peers (Chron-Matched), and their communication age-matched peers (Comm-Matched).

Descriptive Statistics

	Children with CD	Chron-Matched	Comm-Matched
New Method	$M = 54.00$	$M = 49.33$	$M = 51.33$
	$SD = 2.28$	$SD = 2.16$	$SD = 2.28$
	$n = 6$	$n = 6$	$n = 6$
Old Method	$M = 45.92$	$M = 51.17$	$M = 47.41$
	$SD = 2.20$	$SD = 2.14$	$SD = 2.24$
	$n = 6$	$n = 6$	$n = 6$

Analysis of Variance

Source	df	Sums of Squares	Mean Square	F-Ratio	Probability
Group	2	6.51	3.26	0.52	0.60
Method	1	88.67	88.67	14.07	0.0008
Group by Method	2	140.51	70.26	11.15	0.0002
Error	30	189.04	6.30		
Total	35	424.74			

Note: df = degrees of freedom.

2. Select an article that includes quantitative data analysis in the results section. You might select one of the articles below or something on a topic of interest. Make a point to read the results section carefully. What statistical information did the authors report? Descriptive statistics? Inferential statistics? Did the authors use an analysis of variance? If yes, what were the results? How did they present the information from their statistical analysis?

Nonexperimental Research

Archibald, L. M. D., & Gathercole, S. E. (2006). Visuospatial immediate memory in specific language impairment. *Journal of Speech, Language, and Hearing Research, 49,* 265–277.

Bajaj, A. (2007). Analysis of oral narratives of children who stutter and their fluent peers: Kindergarten through second grade. *Clinical Linguistics & Phonetics, 21*(3), 227–245.

Hicks, C. B., & Tharpe, A. M. (2002). Listening effort and fatigue in school-age children with and without hearing loss. *Journal of Speech, Language, and Hearing Research, 45,* 573–584.

Moeller, M. P., Hoover, B., Putnam, C., Arbataitis, K., Bohnenkamp, G., Petersen, B., et al. (2007). Vocalizations of infants with hearing loss compared with infants with normal hearing: Part I. Phonetic development. *Ear and Hearing, 28,* 605–627.

Experimental Research

Almost, D., & Rosenbaum, P. (1998). Effectiveness of speech intervention for phonological disorders: A randomized controlled trial. *Developmental Medicine and Child Neurology, 40*(5), 319–325.

Chisolm, T. H., Abrams, H. B., & McArdle, R. (2004). Short- and long-term outcomes of adult audiological rehabilitation. *Ear and Hearing, 25*(5), 464–477.

Cohen, W., Hodson, A., O'Hare, A., Boyle, J., Durrani, T., McCartney, E., et al. (2005). Effects of computer-based intervention through acoustically modified speech (Fast ForWord) in severe mixed receptive-expressive language impairment: Outcomes from a randomized controlled trial. *Journal of Speech, Language, and Hearing Research, 48*, 715–729.

Doesborgh, S. J., van de Sandt-Koenderman, M. W., Dippel, D. W., van Harskamp, F., Koudstaal, P. J., & Visch-Brink, E. G. (2003). Effects of semantic treatment on verbal communication and linguistic processing in aphasia after stroke: A randomized controlled trial. *Stroke, 35*(1), 141–146.

Ebbels, S. H., van der Lely, H. K., & Dockrell, J. E. (2007). Intervention for verb argument structure in children with persistent SLI: A randomized control trial. *Journal of Speech, Language, and Hearing Research, 50*, 1330–1349.

Harris, V., Onslow, M., Packman, A., Harrison, E., & Menzies, R. (2002). An experimental investigation of the impact of the Lidcombe Program on early stuttering. *Journal of Fluency Disorders, 27*(3), 203–213.

Hesketh, A., Dima, E., & Nelson, V. (2007). Teaching phoneme awareness to pre-literate children with speech disorder: A randomized controlled trial. *International Journal of Language and Communication Disorders, 42*, 251–271.

Rvachew, S., Nowak, M., & Cloutier, G. (2004). Effect of phonemic perception training on the speech production and phonological awareness skills of children with expressive phonological delay. *American Journal of Speech-Language Pathology, 13*, 250–263.

Sapir, S., Spielman, J. L., Ramig, L. O., Story, B. H., & Fox, C. (2007). Effects of intensive voice treatment (the Lee Silverman Voice Treatment [LSVT]) on vowel articulation in dysarthric individuals with idiopathic Parkinson disease: Acoustic and perceptual findings. *Journal of Speech, Language, and Hearing Research, 50*, 899–912,

van Kleeck, A., Vander Woude, J., & Hammett, L. (2006). Fostering literal and inferential language skills in Head Start preschoolers with language impairment using scripted book-sharing discussions. *American Journal of Speech-Language Pathology, 15*, 85–95.

References

American Psychological Association. (2001). *Publication manual of the American Psychological Association* (5th ed.). Washington, DC: Author.

Coladarci, T., Cobb, C. D., Minium, E. W., & Clarke, R. B. (2008). *Fundamentals of statistical reasoning in education* (2nd ed.). Hoboken, NJ: John Wiley & Sons.

DataDesk (version 6.2). (2003). Ithaca, NY: Data Description.

Gibbons, J. D., & Chakraborti, S. (2003). *Nonparametric statistical inference* (4th ed.). Boca Raton, FL: CRC Press-Taylor & Francis Group.

Jacobs, K. W. (1976). A table for the determination of experimentwise error rate (alpha) from independent comparisons. *Educational and Psychological Measurement, 36*, 899–903.

Ottenbacher, K. J. (1986). A quantitative analysis of experimentwise error rates in applied behavioral science research. *Journal of Applied Behavioral Science, 22*, 495–501.

Patten, M. L. (2007). *Understanding research methods: An overview of the essentials* (6th ed.). Glendale, CA: Pyrczak.

Popham, W. J., & Sirotnik, K. A. (1973). *Educational statistics: Use and interpretation* (2nd ed.). New York: Harper and Row.

Pyrczak, F. (2006). *Making sense of statistics: A conceptual overview* (4th ed.). Glendale, CA: Pyrczak.

Rosenthal, R., & Rosnow, R. L. (2008). *Essentials of behavioral research: Methods and data analysis* (3rd ed.). New York: McGraw Hill.

StatSoft, Inc. (2007). *Electronic statistics textbook.* Tulsa, OK: StatSoft. Retrieved March 31, 2008, from http://www.statsoft.com/textbook/stat home.html

Trochim, W. M. K., & Donnelly, J. P. (2007). *The research methods knowledge base* (3rd ed.). Mason, OH: Thomson Custom.

Velleman, P. F. (1997). *DataDesk version 6.0 statistics guide.* Ithaca, NY: Data Description.

Woods, A., Fletcher, P., & Hughes, A. (1986). *Statistics in language studies.* Cambridge, UK: Cambridge University Press.

CHAPTER 10

Research Outcomes: Clinical Guidance, Research Reports

Perhaps the primary reason for professionals in communication sciences and disorders to engage in research is to make certain that their clients receive the best possible audiology and speech-language pathology services (Johnson, 2006). This research might fall under the category of evidence-based practice (EBP) and include a careful search and evaluation of existing research reports to uncover information to guide clinical decisions. Alternatively, this research might fall under the category of original, empirical research and involve gathering new data to answer previously unanswered questions. As we discussed in earlier chapters, the knowledge and skills needed to engage in evidence-based practice and empirical research overlap to a great extent; however, the two forms of research lead to different final products. In EBP research the culminating phases of the investigation include critically evaluating the existing research and considering its appropriateness for your clients and setting (Gallagher, 2002; Johnson, 2006). The research outcome is a clinical decision guided by the best available evidence (American Speech-Language-Hearing Association [ASHA], 2004; Gallagher, 2002), as well as by the clinician's expertise and client/family values (Gallagher, 2002;

Johnson, 2006). In empirical research the final phase is preparation of a research report with the goal of presenting that report at a national or international conference and/or publishing it in a professional journal.

Knowledge Base for Evaluating Clinical Research

Evidence-based practice is an approach to providing professional service that emerged in the field of medicine but subsequently has been incorporated into many areas of professional service, including audiology and speech-language pathology (ASHA, 2004). The approach has been summarized in a series of research steps beginning with formulation of a clinical question, completing a thorough search of professional literature, reviewing and critiquing the identified research, and finally, deciding how to apply the information in your clinical practice and how to evaluate and document your outcomes (Gallagher, 2002; Johnson, 2006).

The goal of EBP is to improve our clinical decision making by reducing overreliance on expert opinion, increasing use of the best available evidence, and integrating use of evidence with clinical expertise and client/family desires and values (ASHA, 2004; Gallagher, 2002). For audiologists and speech-language pathologists to be competent in the process of EBP, they need knowledge of research design to judge the value of the available evidence and information literacy skills to find relevant studies quickly and efficiently (Nail-Chiwetalu & Ratner, 2006; Ratner, 2006). Additionally, they need to include the persons and families who receive services in the decision-making process. This means being able to communicate about "best practice" evidence in language clients and families will understand and having skills to facilitate decision making by consensus and resolving conflicts.

Critical Appraisal

One of the concluding phases in the EBP process involves reading and appraising the identified research. If you were fortunate enough to identify a systematic review or meta-analysis on your topic, you have a single document that lists much of the available research on a topic, includes a review and evaluation of the available studies, and may include a statistical analysis or meta-analysis of the aggregated results across several studies (ASHA, 2008a; Johnson, 2006; Patten, 2007; Trochim & Donnelly, 2007). However, you need to judge the value of even this type of document. Some factors to consider include, first, whether or not the document addresses the actual topic of the search. Search terms, such as *adult, child, speech, language, hearing, treatment, aphasia, voice, fluency or stuttering, phonology, perception*, and so forth, will lead to highly relevant articles as well as to less relevant articles on related topics. For example, if searching for research on treatment of pho-

nological disorders in children, you might need to eliminate studies that addressed phonological or phonemic awareness and literacy skills; similarly, if searching for research on speech perception, the term *speech recognition* might lead to many studies of computer-based speech recognition. An EBP question usually has a specific clinical focus and you need to read and review articles that pertain to that focus (Johnson, 2006).

A second consideration is the source of the review. Some sources are highly regarded professional organizations (ASHA, 2008a; Cochrane Collaboration, n.d.). Other highly regarded sources are peer-reviewed professional journals. Such journals have editorial and review policies and procedures designed to assure that published articles are accurate, complete, and well written. Peer review means submitted manuscripts are carefully read and evaluated by persons who are recognized experts on a topic (Nail-Chiwetalu & Ratner, 2006). Through this process authors often have an opportunity to make corrections and resubmit their manuscripts. Ideally, the final, published article in a peer-reviewed journal should provide valuable information. Information about the review procedures for a particular journal may be included on an editorial page published in each issue of the journal or on the publisher's Web site (e.g., ASHA, 2008b).

A third factor to consider is the date of the review. A review may be well written and published in a credible source but have less value if it is several years old. Research completed and published after the review was finished, often a year or more before its actual publication, would not be included. If you find a relevant but dated systematic review, consider one of the search approaches described in Chapter 4 that allow you to search for articles that cite the report you identified. That way you would be able to find more recent articles, usually on a similar topic, that cite the older review.

If the available evidence on a topic is insufficient for a systematic review, you might have uncovered a few or several studies to read and review yourself. A critical appraisal of research reports often starts with judging the strength of the research design and level of evidence. Thus, knowing what constitutes a strong research design is essential in the EBP process. The information in Chapter 5 and Chapter 6, and in particular Table 6-5, should be useful in identifying research designs and levels of evidence. In a well-written research report the authors should state the type of research design they employed. For treatment studies, the strongest designs are variations of randomized group designs such as a pretest-posttest randomized control group design. In this kind of research the groups are usually experimental treatment and no-treatment control groups or experimental treatment and traditional treatment groups. A single group pretest-posttest design is a weak design and inappropriate for establishing treatment effectiveness. Ideally, peer-reviewed journals would not publish such studies, although you may find this kind of information presented at some professional conferences or included in self-published reports.

Although determining the research design and level of evidence for a research report is a crucial, and often the beginning, step in critical appraisal, additional factors are important as well. Even in randomized control studies some additional characteristics may strengthen the validity of the evidence. One of these characteristics is whether or not those who made observations, completed assessments, and analyzed the data knew the group membership.

When researchers who obtain measurements and analyze data know whether or not participants received the experimental or control treatment, they might even inadvertently bias the measurement and analysis process. When those involved in measurement and analysis do not know who was in the experimental and control groups, they are "blinded" to group membership (ASHA, 2004; Gillam & Gillam, 2006; Schardt & Mayer, 2004).

Another factor to consider is how participants were recruited for the study. In a randomized control study, assignment to groups obviously is random, but the sample might or might not be a random sample. The evidence is stronger if the researchers had many possible participants and randomly selected the groups from this larger set. A related factor is the size of the sample. Davidow, Bothe, and Bramlett (2006) suggested 10 participants per group as a minimum sample size for research in fluency disorders. However, if the expected difference is small but important, even 10 persons per group would be inadequate (Rosenthal & Rosnow, 2008). Other factors being equal, a large sample is more representative of a population than a small sample (Patten, 2007).

Another issue to consider is whether or not any participants dropped out over the course of the study (Davidow et al., 2006; Schardt & Mayer, 2004). The loss of participants could affect the results of a study if the loss occurred due to systematic rather than random factors. For example, if some participants experienced little or no benefit from an experimental treatment, they might drop out of the study. This would leave only those persons who experienced positive outcomes for the posttest measurement and data analysis and would make the treatment look more effective than it actually was. Usually when loss of participants occurs, researchers include some explanation of this and even a follow-up analysis to determine if those who dropped out differed from those who finished the study in some systematic way.

Another question to consider when evaluating an experimental treatment study is who provided the treatment. Did the researchers employ one therapist or several and what were their qualifications (Davidow et al., 2006)? If only one audiologist or speech-language pathologist provided the treatment and it proved to be effective, that result might be due to the qualities of a uniquely talented clinician. One the other hand, if a promising treatment approach proved to be ineffective, that result could have occurred because of some limitation in the clinician's skills. A study in which several well-trained clinicians provided the treatment would be stronger than one in which a single, perhaps inexperienced clinician provided the treatment. One way that researchers might address the issue of quality and consistency of the treatment would be to monitor and analyze treatment delivery and include that information in the research report.

The adequacy of the dependent variables or outcome measures is another consideration (Gillam & Gillam, 2006; McCauley, Weston, Rvachew, Williams, & Weiss, 2004). Audiologists and speech-language pathologists, through their clinical training and experience, are well qualified to evaluate formal and informal measures of treatment progress. The expectation is that researchers will select outcome measures that have proven reliability and validity. Alternately, if the researchers use a novel measure that has not been well studied, they should include information about reliability and validity in the research report. Another question about outcome measures concerns the extent to which the researchers assessed generalization outside the experimental setting or included measures that addressed improvement in social participation (McCauley et al., 2004). A final consideration is whether the researchers obtained both short-term and long-term outcome measures (Davidow et al., 2006). Many otherwise well-designed studies have limited outcome data consisting of treatment probes obtained in the experimental setting shortly after the conclusion of treatment.

Although randomized group designs provide the strongest evidence, practical limitations sometimes force researchers to use quasi-experimental or single participant research designs. When the design is a quasi-experimental, nonrandom control group design, including a pretest is essential to establish that treatment and control groups were similar at the start of the study (Schardt & Mayer, 2004). Otherwise, the researchers will not know whether to attribute differences observed at the end of the study to treatment effects or preexisting group differences. In single participant research, we need to consider the strength of the design as well. The simplest single participant design is a baseline and treatment design. Such a design is seldom adequate for experimental purposes and researchers usually adopt a stronger design, such as a treatment replication design and/or a multiple baseline across participants design. If the single participant research involves comparing more than one treatment, the researchers need to consider the possibility of order of treatment effects. Recruiting four or more participants and randomly assigning them to different treatment orders is one way for researchers to address the issue of order in single participant designs.

The source of a research report is an important consideration as well. If you found an unpublished research report on the Internet, you should question why the authors never published the study. Certainly authors have good reasons for generating a self-published report and not submitting it for peer review; however, some self-published reports are of low quality. Generally, reports from peer-reviewed sources are more trustworthy than those from personal Web sites or nonreviewed publications (Nail-Chiwetalu & Ratner, 2006). Some additional factors to consider in evaluating a study are the breadth of evidence and the source of the evidence. Recall that the highest level of evidence is a meta-analysis or systematic review and that you need several studies on the same topic to prepare this type of document. When evaluating the "body of evidence" for a particular treatment, you need to consider how many studies are available, whether these studies provide conflicting or converging evidence (ASHA, 2004), and who conducted the study and wrote the research report. A body of evidence from multiple researchers, persons other than those who first developed an approach, and multiple treatment sites would be much stronger than evidence from a single research group (Nail-Chiwetalu & Ratner, 2006; Ratner, 2006). The various criteria for appraising clinical research are summarized in Table 10–1.

How Applicable Are the Findings

Audiologists and speech-language pathologists ultimately must decide whether or not research findings apply to their clients and clinical settings. Even information from a well-designed study may have limited value if the participants in the study and your clients have different characteristics. Similarly, the findings may have little practical importance if the intensity of treatment, type of treatment, or required equipment is unique to the research setting. Researchers should report detailed information about their participants, including information about ages, gender, type and severity of disorder, cultural, ethnic and linguistic background, educational level, family incomes, and so forth (Gillam & Gillam, 2006). Some of this information will be more important for certain types of experimental treatments than others, but having a detailed description of participants is a crucial section in any research report. Similarly, professionals conducting EBP research need detailed descriptions of the treatment procedures and settings in order to judge how similar the research setting was to their clinical setting.

After completing a literature search and reading and evaluating several research reports, audiologists and speech-language

---

Table 10–1. Summary of criteria for critical appraisal of a research report

1. Purpose or focus of the study
2. Basic research design
   - Randomized group design — If yes, what type?
   - Quasi-experimental group design — If yes, what type?
   - Single participant design — If yes, what type?
   - Case study — If yes, what type?
   - Other — Specify

continued

Table 10–1. *continued*

3. Other design features
   - Pretest   If yes, were participants similar?
   - Long-term posttest   Briefly describe
   - Blinding for outcome measurement

4. Participants
   - Age   Briefly describe
   - Diagnosis, if relevant   Briefly describe
   - Gender   Briefly describe
   - Cultural and linguistic background   Briefly describe
   - Random assignment to groups
   - Random selection   If not randomly selected, briefly
                                                describe participant recruitment
   - Number of participants in each group
   - Participant loss   If yes, did the authors include an
                                                explanation?

5. Treatment dependability
   - One or several clinicians
   - Qualifications of the clinician(s)
   - Procedures to monitor treatment   Briefly describe

6. Outcome measures
   - Tests with known reliability and validity
   - Informal or unique measures   If yes, did the authors include
                                                information about reliability and validity?
   - Generalization measures   Briefly describe

7. Source of the report
   - Peer-reviewed
   - Publication, but not peer-reviewed
   - Presentation at peer-reviewed
     conference
   - Presentation at conference, but not
     peer-reviewed
   - Web site   If yes, is it a reputable source?
   - Other

8. Body of evidence
   - Multiple studies   If yes, are findings similar or conflicting?
   - Multiple treatment centers
   - Researchers other than originators

pathologists need to make a decision about adopting a particular treatment approach. One aspect of this decision is weighing the costs and potential benefits of the new treatment (Johnson, 2006). Costs might include greater demands on the clinicians' time to prepare and provide the new treatment. Other costs are more direct, such as paying for specialized training required to deliver the new treatment. A treatment with high costs would need to show substantial benefit to justify its adoption.

Additional factors in deciding how to apply findings from EBP research are the client's and family's opinions and values. Families sometimes hear about and desire certain treatment approaches because of information they obtained from friends and acquaintances or from nonreviewed information sources such as the Internet. Audiologists and speech-language pathologists need to weigh the desires of the client and family against the strength of the empirical evidence. If strong evidence is available that is consistent with client and family desires, then no conflict exists. However, if strong evidence is available that goes counter to the family's choices, professionals ethically need to recommend and implement the most effective treatment. In this case, the audiologist or speech-language pathologist needs to communicate with the client and family about what the evidence shows and facilitate resolution of any conflicts that may arise. Although the audiologists' or speech-language pathologists' expertise is always an important factor in clinical decision making, this expertise is even more important when the evidence is unclear. Clinicians still need to decide how best to serve a client even in the face of limited or conflicting evidence. In such cases they need to choose based on

their own expertise, carefully monitor the client's progress, and make adjustments to the treatment approach as needed.

Significance of Results and Effect Size

Researchers almost always include some type of inferential statistical analysis when conducting a group comparison study. Recall that the role of inferential statistics is to provide an estimate of the probability of error in saying that two groups are different. An error would be concluding that two groups are different, when in the actual population the two groups are similar. When researchers report that the difference between groups was significant, they are saying that the probability of error was acceptably low, usually a less than 5 in 100 chance. However, a difference between groups can be statistically significant without being practically important. For example, small mean difference could be statistically significant if the comparison groups were large enough. Measures of effect size are one way to convey the practical significance of an observed difference.

Several different measures are available for looking at magnitude of effects and effect size (Patten, 2007; Trochim & Donnelly, 2007). One of the most common measures, *Cohen's d*, converts the mean difference between groups into a standard unit of difference based on standard deviation (Patten, 2007). To compute this measure you need to know the means and standard deviations for each group. Cohen's d is calculated as follows: $M_1 - M_2$/pooled standard deviation[1] (Hargrove, 2002; Patten, 2007). Let's consider the following example.

---

[1]The formula for computing a pooled standard deviation is available from several sources (e.g., Hargrove, 2002; Patten, 2007; Yampolsky & Matthies, 2002). The formula is: square root of $((n_1 - 1) sd_1^2 + (n_2 - 1) sd_2^2 /(n_1 + n_2 - 2))$.

A group of audiologists and speech-language pathologists conducted a posttest-only study with randomized experimental treatment and control groups. The experimental group received a M of 59.6 with a SD of 13.4, whereas the control group had a M of 49.6 with a SD of 12.9. Each group had 25 participants. Thus, the pooled standard deviation was the square root of $(25 - 1)13.4^2 + (25 - 1)12.9^2/(25 + 25 - 2)$ or 13.15; and the effect size represented by Cohen's d was $(59.6 - 49.6)/13.15$ or 0.76. Cohen (as cited in Patten, 2007) suggested that a d of 0.20 corresponded to a small treatment effect, a d of 0.50 corresponded to a medium treatment effect, and a d of 0.80 corresponded to a large treatment effect.

Another option for conveying effect size includes an *effect size r*, which is similar to a Pearson r (Meline & Paradiso, 2003; Patten, 2007). Like the Pearson r the values of an effect size r range from 0.0 to ± 1.00. Patten (2007) noted that an effect size r could be estimated if you know Cohen's d using the formula: $r_{es} = d$ divided by the square root of $(d^2 + 4)$. Patten also noted r_{es} is easier to interpret when you convert it to an r^2 and multiply r^2 by 100. This yields a number similar to a coefficient of determination, as discussed in Chapter 9. Thus, for the example we calculated above, with a d of 0.76, the $r_{es} = 0.76$/square root of $(0.76^2 + 4)$ or $r_{es} = 0.34$ and $r^2 = 0.116$, for a percentage of 11.6%.

One additional effect size measure is *number needed to treat* (Trochim & Donnelly, 2007). This is an effect size measure often used in the field of medicine. It reflects how many patients doctors would need to treat before they found someone who experienced a benefit from a treatment. For example, you might compare a new medication and a placebo and ask how many patients needed to take the new medicine before someone experienced an improvement. A lower number needed to treat is better; thus, a new medicine that is effective for 1 out of 3 patients is better than a new medicine that is effective for 1 out of 10 patients. Although effect size measures were seldom reported for older studies, new research reports should include this information because reporting effect sizes is one component in current standards for research publications (ASHA, 2008b; Consolidated Standards of Reporting Trials [CONSORT] Group, 2001).

Given the level of knowledge and skills needed to participate in EBP research, many might wonder why this concept has become firmly established across many professions. The answer involves weighing the costs in terms of training and time against the benefits. A few of the many benefits of evidence-based practice include: (a) improved services for the persons audiologists and speech-language pathologists serve professionally (ASHA, 2004), (b) increased opportunities for research funding by improving our professions' standing in the research community, (c) increased public and private support for our services by using evidence that documents its effectiveness, and (d) enhanced ability to respond to questions about the cost and effectiveness of our services. Although individual audiologists and speech-language pathologists need knowledge and skills to participate in evidence-based practice research, this type of research is not ideally an individual effort. The quality and availability of EBP research will be greater through collective and collaborative efforts (Johnson, 2006).

Reporting Research Findings

In empirical research the final phase is preparation and dissemination of a research report. Most research reports follow a similar structure with regard to content.

A well-written report includes: (a) a title that reflects the subject matter of the study; (b) a brief abstract that summarizes the purpose, methods, and results of the study; (c) an introduction and review of previous literature; (d) a methods section with information about participants, instrumentation and procedures, and data analysis; (e) a results section; (f) a discussion section; and (g) references (American Psychological Association [APA], 2001, 2005; Patten, 2007; Trochim & Donnelly, 2007).

Components of a Research Report

The *title* of a research report might be approximately 10 to 15 words long and conveys the essence of the study. A good title usually conveys what actions occurred during the study, such as investigating a relationship, identifying characteristics, or comparing treatments, what the major variables were, and who participated in the study. The *abstract* for a research report is a short synopsis of the content of the entire article. An abstract might range from 100 to 150 words, and some publications have specific guidelines regarding the length of an abstract. The content of the abstract usually includes a statement of purpose, a brief description of the participants, the most important information about instrumentation and procedures, and a brief summary of the most important findings (Patten, 2007; Trochim & Donnelly, 2007). Recently, some journals have adopted a *structured abstract* as a requirement for published articles. Structured abstracts are easy to recognize because you see headings associated with the major parts of the abstract such as Objective, Methods, Results, and Conclusions (Bayley & Eldredge, 2005).[2]

The first section in the main body of a research report is the introduction and review of literature. This section seldom has a section heading, except in longer documents such as theses and dissertations. Often researchers begin a paper with a general statement of purpose or the issue under investigation. The major portion of this first section is a review of important prior work on the topic (APA, 2001). This prior work might take the form of discussions of the theory that is being tested, brief summaries of previous, related research, and a critique of previous research focusing on conflicting evidence and missing information. The literature review typically ends with the authors' reasons for conducting their research, along with an explicit statement of purpose or a set of research questions (Patten, 2007). In most published research reports the review of literature has a relatively narrow focus and does not include general background information that most persons in the field would know. At the same time the review of literature must be up-to-date and cover the primary topics in a thorough manner.

The Methods section follows the review of literature and statement of research questions. This section has subsections such as participants, instrumentation, procedures, and data analysis. The participants section should include a detailed description of participants with information such as age, speech, language, and hearing abilities, educational status, cultural and linguistic background, native language, and so forth. This section should include information about

---

[2]For examples of structured abstracts, you might examine research reports published from 2006 forward in journals such as the *American Journal of Speech-Language Pathology*, *American Journal of Audiology*, and *Journal of Speech-Language-Hearing Research*. You might find examples of unstructured abstracts for comparison in issues of these journals published prior to 2005 or in other journals such as *Journal of the American Academy of Audiology*, *Journal of Fluency Disorders*, and *Journal of Voice*.

how the researchers recruited their participants and procedures for selecting the samples and for assigning participants to groups. The instrumentation section includes a description of measurement tools such as formal tests, questionnaires, and laboratory equipment. This section also should include information about the reliability and validity of the measures employed in the study (Trochim & Donnelly, 2007). The procedures section might also be called design and procedures (Trochim & Donnelly, 2007). This section will include information about the basic design, such as pretest-posttest randomized control group design, multiple baseline across subjects design, or nonexperimental qualitative case study. In addition, the researchers should include information about how frequently they saw the participants, how long the sessions were, who actually administered the treatments or other experimental procedures, and a detailed description of the treatments. The final subsection under Methods is often a data analysis and reliability section.

The next section in a research report is a Results section. In quantitative research, this section presents both descriptive and inferential statistics. The results reported typically relate directly to the research questions and research design. Thus, if the investigation involved a comparison of two measures, readers will expect to see some type of correlation analysis in the results. On the other hand, if the investigation involved determining differences between three or more groups, readers will expect to see some type of analysis of variance. Patten (2007) recommended reporting descriptive information first, and then the results of any inferential statistical tests. When a study has several groups, researchers often present their findings in tables. However, when reporting the results, just stating that the results are shown in Table X is insufficient. Writers should also provide a brief verbal description of the main points shown in the table (Patten, 2007).

The results section in a qualitative research report often begins with a statement of the method of data analysis. The content generally is verbal in nature with few if any numbers. The nature of the data in qualitative research might be a series of "themes" that emerged from the researchers' analysis (Patten, 2007). In addition to these themes, researchers usually include verbatim quotes from interview transcripts and/or detailed descriptions of events and situations that represent the themes.

The fourth section in a research report is the Discussion section, which sometimes is called Discussion and Conclusions, or Discussion and Summary. The discussion usually includes a restatement of the findings without the numerical data. One way to structure a discussion is to include sections that address each of the research questions, either providing an answer to the question, or if the results were ambiguous, explaining that aspect. Authors usually describe how their findings related to previous, similar research on the topic. This might include explicitly noting when findings agree and when they conflict with prior research. If the researchers uncovered conflicting evidence, they usually consider possible explanations for the difference. If the authors presented possible theoretical implications in their review of literature, the discussion section should include an explanation of how the findings relate to theory as well. Usually toward the end of a discussion section authors include information about possible weaknesses in their research, either because of design limitations or because of unanticipated factors that emerged over the course of the study (Patten, 2007). They also consider possible avenues for future research on the topic.

The final section of the research report is the References section. This section includes all the works cited in the paper, including previous research reports, books, chapters in books, documents from Web sites, and so forth. The list of references should only include works actually cited in the paper and no additional items. The list is organized by authors' last names and date of publication. Some research reports include an Appendix, which is an optional section. Authors might decide to include an appendix to provide a lengthy document that might disrupt the flow of ideas in the main body of the manuscript. An appendix might include items such as a questionnaire, a detailed treatment protocol, or a verbatim transcript of an interview.

Writing Guidelines and Writing Style

Most journal publications have editorial guidelines regarding the content, style, and format of manuscripts. In the field of communication sciences and disorders, many publications have adopted American Psychological Association (APA) publication guidelines. These content and style guidelines are presented in depth in the *Publication Manual of the American Psychological Association, Fifth Edition* (APA, 2001) and in a more concise format in *Concise Rules of APA Style* (APA, 2005). The APA style manuals provide guidance on how to write in a clear and concise manner, how to cite sources in the body of your paper, how to organize information in tables and figures, how to report statistical and other numerical information, and how to format entries in a reference list.

When writing a research report, a good strategy is to focus on communicating about the research, rather than on writing in an impressive and entertaining way. Highly regarded research writing is clear, concise, and to the point (Meline & Paradiso, 2003).

The APA (2001, 2005) publication manuals provide considerable writing guidance. When the emphasis is on communication, writers strive to present information in a parallel and consistent way to facilitate comprehension. Understanding information in a list is easier if all of the items start with the same syntactic form. For example, if authors wanted to list a series of actions, they might adopt an infinitive form and begin each item in the list with *to + verb* (e.g., to identify, to select, to evaluate, to decide, and so forth). Similarly, authors should use a single tense throughout certain sections of the paper. APA guidelines suggest staying in past tense for the review of literature, methods, and results section, all of which report completed phases of the research. On the other hand, authors should use present tense in the discussion and conclusions as a way to encourage readers to reflect on the findings with them.

Authors also should use language that ties related ideas together but need to be careful to choose the appropriate linking words (APA, 2001, 2002). Many of us have written sentences such as, "Persons with communication disorders performed better on task A, *while* persons with normal communication performed better on Task B." The intent of this sentence is to contrast the performance of the two groups. However, the transition word *while* has a temporal meaning and literally means doing something at the same time. A better choice of transition word when trying to communicate a contrast is *whereas* or *however*. Similarly, writers sometimes use the word *since* in place of *because*. However, these two words have specific uses. The word *since* conveys a temporal relationship, whereas the word *because* conveys a causal relationship.

In research writing straightforward, relatively short sentences are preferable to lengthy sentences that incorporate many modifiers or link too many ideas together.

Similarly, active voice is preferable to passive voice. Many of us adopt a passive voice to avoid talking about ourselves when we write. For example, I might write, "The participants were tested three times during the study." However, APA guidelines advise using first person to improve the strength and clarity of writing. Therefore, I should write, "I tested the participants three times during the study," (or "We tested . . . " if the research was conducted by more than one person).

Other important guidelines in the APA style manuals address how to refer to persons. One key point is to refer to persons in a specific rather than abstract way (e.g., write about infants, children, persons age 20 to 25, or women age 50 to 65, rather than the "subjects"). A second key point is to strive to put person first rather than characteristics such as disability, age, income level, and so forth. A careful author describes participants as *10 children with specific language impairment, 20 adults with functional voice disorders*, or *10 adults, age 40-65, with moderate-to-severe hearing impairment*. The APA manuals also are extremely useful for those who are uncertain about punctuation and grammatical usage.

APA style includes specific guidelines regarding how to cite sources in the body of your paper and how to format entries in a reference list. A few of the most common examples include:

- Citing a single source by one or two authors
  - In the body of a sentence: Trochim and Donnelly (2007) stated that research design is an important topic.
  - In parentheses at the end of a sentence: Research design is an important topic (Trochim & Donnelly, 2007).
- Citing a single source by three or more authors
  - On first use: Davidow, Bothe, and Bramlett (2003)
  - On subsequent uses: Davidow et al. (2003)
- Citing several sources
  - In parentheses at the end of a sentence: Research design is an important topic (Patten, 2007; Rosenthal & Rosnow, 2008; Trochim & Donnelly, 2007).

In APA style, authors cite sources by author and date and list multiple sources alphabetically. When an article has three or more authors, the citation is shortened after the first mention. There are many variations on authorship and the APA publication manuals include many examples of citing these variations.

The reference list includes an entry for each citation in the text of the manuscript. APA publication guidelines also specify how to format different types of sources in the reference list. Some common sources are journal articles, books, chapters in edited books, and documents from Web sites. The format for each of these sources is illustrated below:

- Journal article:
  Chisolm, T. H., Abrams, H. B., & McArdle, R. (2004). Short- and long-term outcomes of adult audiological rehabilitation. *Ear and Hearing, 25*(5), 464-477.
- Book:
  Trochim, W. M. K., & Donnelly, J. P. (2007). *The research methods knowledge base* (3rd ed.). Mason, OH: Thomson Custom Publishing.
- Chapter in an edited book:

Kratochwill, T. R. (1992). Single-case research design and analysis: An overview. In T. R. Kratochwill & J. R. Level (Eds.), *Single-case research design and analysis: New directions for psychology and education* (pp. 1–14). Hillsdale, NJ: Lawrence Erlbaum Associates.

■ Document from a Web site: American Speech-Language-Hearing Association. (2004). *Evidence-based practice in communication disorders: An introduction* [Technical report]. Retrieved January 3, 2007, from http://www.asha.org/docs/html/TR2004-00001.html

Each of the sources above was listed by author and date. The Web site document was authored by an organization, and other variations on authorship are covered in the APA manuals. Each of the listings also had a title and information about the source of the document—the journal, the publisher, or the Web address.

Authors who want guidance regarding the recommended content for research reports have several sources to consult. Recent group initiatives resulted in reporting guidelines for randomized clinical trials, nonrandomized research designs, and studies of diagnostic tests (Bossuyt et al., 2003; CONSORT Group, 2001; Des Jarlais, Lyles, Crepaz, & the TREND Group, 2004). Each of these documents includes information about recommended content for various sections of research reports, including background information, methods and participants, results and data analysis, and discussion.

Disseminating Research Findings

When authors prepare a research report, they usually have a plan for disseminating the information. Their options include publication in a peer-reviewed journal, a presentation at a professional conference, and self-published reports. Generally, articles in peer-reviewed journals have higher status because these articles have met standards set by the journal editorial board. Peer review includes reading and evaluation of manuscripts prior to publication by persons with expertise on the topic. The field of communication sciences and disorders has many peer-reviewed journals, some published by professional organizations such as the American Speech-Language-Hearing Association and the American Academy of Audiology (AAA), and others from private publishers. In some fields of study, Web-based journals are emerging as an alternative to traditional print media, and many of these have editorial policies that require peer review prior to publication.

Another option for disseminating information is a presentation at a professional conference. Some conference presentations are poster sessions or visual presentations of a research report, with large type designed to be read at a distance, extensive use of charts and graphs, and limited text (e.g., bulleted points or brief figure captions). The poster usually includes all components of a research report including introduction and research questions, methods and participants, results, and discussion. However, the introduction and discussion tend to be brief and authors emphasize their methods and results.

Some conference programs also include technical sessions and technical papers. A technical paper is a relatively brief oral presentation, often accompanied by a few slides depicting key information. Like poster sessions, researchers making oral presentations usually include a brief introduction, spend most of their time explaining the methods and results, and end with a brief discussion. Typically, a technical session groups together several papers on related topics.

Some professional conferences also include research seminars in their schedule. Seminars are longer sessions often lasting 1½ to 2 hours. Researchers who present during a research seminar often have conducted several related studies on a topic and present the aggregated findings of this research. The longer format of a research seminar allows the presenters to spend more time discussing theoretical issues and the implications of their findings.

Students in master's and doctoral level graduate programs often conduct empirical research and prepare a thesis or dissertation. Theses and dissertations have an alternate distribution model. Most are housed in the libraries of the universities where they were produced. Doctoral dissertations and some master's theses also are distributed via the ProQuest Dissertations and Theses database (ProQuest, 2008). The ProQuest databases are searchable and allow general access to abstracts and provide a purchase option for most of the documents in the database. Dissertations and theses undergo a review process that is similar to peer review. Graduate students who are completing a dissertation or thesis have a committee of faculty who have expertise related to the topic of the research. This faculty committee must approve the document before it is distributed.

A final option for disseminating a research report is to generate and distribute a self-published report. With an increase in Internet usage, the usual way to distribute a self-published report is via a Web site. Some of these reports are distributed as a requirement of a research grant. The individuals who received a government grant to fund their research sometimes are obligated to prepare and disseminate a report in a way that makes it generally available with no fee. Another reason for disseminating a self-published report is that the authors were unable to find a professional journal that would publish the study. Ratner (2006) noted that research journals often have a bias toward publishing only studies with significant findings. Researchers could conduct a well-designed study and prepare a clearly written report but find that they cannot publish it because their findings were not statistically significant. Ratner noted clinicians need to know about treatment approaches that did not work as well as those that did. Thus, researchers who distribute self-published reports may be providing important information. However, self-published reports usually have not gone through a formal review process, and clinicians and researchers need to be careful when using the information from such sources.

Summary

Research in the field of communication sciences and disorders encompasses both investigation of the existing research base to find answers to clinical questions, called evidence-based practice, and original empirical research to investigate unanswered questions that are theoretical and/or clinical in nature. EBP begins with formulation of a focused clinical question and progresses to a search of professional literature, to review and critical appraisal of the identified research, and finally to a decision about how to apply the information in professional practice. The process of critical appraisal requires knowledge of research design, the ability to judge the credibility of a source, knowledge of reliable and valid approaches to assessing outcomes, the ability to discuss evidence with clients and families, and the ability to determine if the available evidence applies to one's clients and setting.

When reading research reports, audiologists and speech-language pathologists need to consider the practical significance of the findings. A difference between groups can be statistically significant without being practically important. One way to determine practical significance is to apply a measure of effect size. Ideally, authors should include an effect size measure along with other statistical information in the results section of a research report. If the authors reported their means and standard deviation, you also could compute some effect size measures on your own.

In empirical research the final phase is preparation and dissemination of a research report. Authors might publish their findings in a peer-reviewed journal or present a paper at a professional conference. In some circumstances, such as when a study did not yield statistically significant findings, they might consider distributing a self-published report. Although the various forms of information dissemination differ, the various report types usually have similar sections: a title, abstract, introduction and review of literature, methods, results, discussion and conclusions, and references. Usually peer-reviewed journals contain the highest quality research reports, because these journals have a process in which all manuscripts are read and evaluated by persons with expertise on the topic prior to publication.

Review Questions

1. What step comes first in evidence-based practice research?
   a. Completing a thorough literature search
   b. Deciding how to use your findings
   c. Formulating a focused clinical question
   d. Reading and evaluating research reports

2. What phase in evidence-based practice research involves reading existing research reports and using your knowledge of research design, measurement, and so on, to evaluate those reports?

3. Explain why articles published in peer-reviewed journals have higher status than self-published reports.

4. Explain why blinding is a desirable feature in treatment studies.

5. Identify two reasons why statistically significant differences might not be practically important in a clinical setting.

6. Explain why a body of evidence from different researchers and different clinical settings is stronger than a single randomized clinical trial.

7. List seven sections that are included in most research reports.

8. What is a structured abstract?

9. Where will you find the formal statement of purpose and/or research questions in most research reports?

10. For each of the sentence pairs below, identify the one that best meets the writing guideline.

Presents information in a parallel form:

a. The participants most often reported writing for program information, the Web sites for each program, contacts with previous graduates, and receiving information from the ASHA Council on Academic Affairs.

b. The participants most often reported receiving information from written contacts with each program, the Web sites for each program, their contacts with previous graduates, and the ASHA Council on Academic Affairs.

Uses affect/effect correctly:

a. The high frequency distractor signal effected the results for both children and adults.

b. The high frequency distractor signal affected the results for both children and adults.

Uses the most appropriate linking term:

a. The 6-year-old children performed significantly better under condition A, whereas the 9-year-old children performed significantly better under condition B.

b. The 6-year-old children performed significantly better under condition A, while the 9-year-old children performed significantly better under condition B.

Uses active voice:

a. Smith and Jones (2001) conducted a study to validate the new test procedure.

b. A study was conducted by Smith and Jones (2001) to validate the new test procedure.

Uses the "person first" rule:

a. As shown in Table 1, the aphasics had higher scores in the experimental treatment.

b. As shown in Table 1, individuals with aphasia had higher mean scores in the experimental treatment.

11. Many journals in the field of communication sciences and disorders use the same writing and style guidelines. What is the source of these guidelines?

12. Each of the following entries in a reference list has an error. Identify the error and correct it.

Blackstock, J., and Miller, L. (1992). The impact of new information technology on young children's symbol-weaving efforts. *Computers and Education, 18,* 209–221.

Clements, D. H., & Nastasi, B. K. (1993). Electronic media and early childhood education. In B. Spodek (Ed.), *Handbook of research on the education of young children.* New York: Macmillan (pp. 251–274).

Haugland, S. W. (1995). Classroom Activities Provide Important Support to Children's Computer Experiences. *Early Childhood Education Journal, 23,* 99–100.

Haugland, S. W., & Wright, J. L. (1997). *Young children and technology: A world of discovery.* Allyn and Bacon: Boston.

Shriberg et al. (1989). Tabletop versus microcomputer-assisted speech management: Stabilization phase. *Journal of Speech and Hearing Disorders, 54,* 233–248.

Learning Activities

1. Identify a research report on a topic of interest. Read this article and prepare a brief summary like the ones you have read in the professional literature. You might find the following Web sites helpful in preparing your summary.

   Purdue OWL. (2006, September 10). Quoting, paraphrasing, and summarizing. In *The Purdue Online Writing Lab*. Retrieved November 19, 2007, from http://owl.english.purdue.edu/owl/resource/563/01/

   Purdue OWL. (2007, October 11). Paraphrase: Write it in your own words. In *The Purdue Online Writing Lab*. Retrieved November 19, 2007, from http://owl.english.purdue.edu/owl/resource/563/02/

   UW-Madison Writing Center. (2006). *Writer's handbook*. Retrieved November 19, 2007, from http://www.wisc.edu/writing/Handbook/index.html

2. Use the information in Table 10–1 to complete a critical appraisal of a research report on a treatment topic. If you read a treatment-related report for activity 1, you could use the same report. Otherwise, you could identify another report that covers a treatment approach that you find interesting.

References

American Psychological Association. (2001). *Publication manual of the American Psychological Association* (5th ed.). Washington, DC: Author.

American Psychological Association. (2005). *Concise rules of APA style*. Washington, DC: Author.

American Speech-Language-Hearing Association. (2004). *Evidence-based practice in communication disorders: An introduction* [Technical report]. Retrieved January 3, 2007, from http://www.asha.org/docs/html/TR2004-00001.html

American Speech-Language-Hearing Association. (2008a). *Compendium of EBP guidelines and systematic reviews*. Retrieved May 2, 2008, from http://www.asha.org/members/ebp/compendium/

American Speech-Language-Hearing Association. (2008b). *Manuscript submissions & instructions for authors*. Retrieved May 2, 2008, from http://www.asha.org/about/publications/journal-abstracts/submissions/

American Speech-Language-Hearing Association. (n.d.). *ASHA publications*. Retrieved January 7, 2008, from http://www.asha.org/about/publications/

Bayley, L., & Eldredge, J. D. (2005). The structured abstract: An essential tool for researchers. *MLA Research Section*. Retrieved May 2, 2008, from http://research.mlanet.org/structured_abstract.html

Bossuyt, P. M., Reitsma, J. B., Bruns, D. E., Gatsonis, C. A., Glasziou, P. P., Irwig, L. M., et al. for the STARD Group. (2003). Towards complete and accurate reporting of studies of diagnostic accuracy: The STARD initiative [Electronic version]. *American Journal of Clinical Pathology, 119*, 18–22.

The Cochrane Collaboration. (n.d.). Retrieved May 2, 2008, from http://www.cochrane.org/

Consolidated Standards of Reporting Trials (CONSORT) Group. (2001). *CONSORT statement 2001—checklist: Items to include when reporting a randomized trial*. Retrieved on May 5, 2008, from http://www.consort-statement.org/mod_product/uploads/CONSORT%202001%20checklist.pdf

Davidow, J. H., Bothe, A. K., & Bramlett, R. E. (2006). The Stuttering Treatment Research Evaluation and Assessment Tool (STREAT): Evaluating treatment research as part of evidence-based practice. *American Journal of Speech-Language Pathology, 15*, 126–141.

Des Jarlais, D. C., Lyles, C., Crepaz, N., & the TREND Group. (2004). Improving the reporting quality of nonrandomized evaluations of behavioral and public health interventions: The TREND statement [Electronic version]. *American Journal of Public Health, 94*(3), 361–366.

Gallagher, T. M. (2002). Evidence-based practice: Applications to speech-language pathology. *Perspectives on Language Learning and Education, 9*(1), 2–5.

Gillam, S. L., & Gillam, R. B. (2006). Making evidence-based decisions about child language intervention in schools. *Language, Speech, and Hearing Services in Schools, 37*, 304–315.

Hargrove, P. (2002, October). Evidence-based practice tutorial #3: Identifying the magnitude of the effect. *Perspectives on Language Learning and Education, 9*(3), 34–36.

Johnson, C. J. (2006). Getting started in evidence-based practice for childhood speech-language disorders. *American Journal of Speech-Language Pathology, 15*, 20–35.

McCauley, R., Weston, A., Rvachew, S., Williams, L., & Weiss, A. (2004, November,). *Evidence-based practice and speech sound disorders: The why? And the how?* Paper presented at the annual convention of the American Speech-Language-Hearing Association, Philadelphia, PA.

Meline, T., & Paradiso, T. (2003). Evidence-based practice in schools: Evaluating research and reducing barriers. *Language, Speech, and Hearing Services in Schools, 34*, 273–283.

Nail-Chiwetalu, B. J., & Ratner, N. B. (2006). Information literacy for speech-language pathologists: A key to evidence-based practice. *Language, Speech, and Hearing Services in Schools, 37*, 157–167.

Patten, M. L. (2007). *Understanding research methods: An overview of the essentials* (6th ed.). Glendale, CA: Pyrczak.

ProQuest. (2008). Retrieved May 5, 2008, from http://proquest.umi.com/login

Ratner, N. B. (2006). Evidence-based practice: An examination of its ramifications for the practice of speech-language pathology. *Language, Speech, and Hearing Services in Schools, 37*, 257–267.

Rosenthal, R., & Rosnow, R. L. (2008). *Essentials of behavioral research: Methods and data analysis* (3rd ed.). New York: McGraw Hill.

Schardt, C., & Mayer, J. (2004). *Introduction to evidence-based medicine.* Duke University Medical Center Library and Health Sciences Library, UNC-Chapel Hill. Retrieved January 8, 2007, from http://www.hsl.unc.edu/services/tutorials/ebm/index.htm

Trochim, W. M. K., & Donnelly, J. P. (2007). *The research methods knowledge base* (3rd ed.). Mason, OH: Thomson Custom.

Yampolsky, S. A., & Matthies, M. L. (2002). Evidence-based practice in speech-language pathology. *Perspectives on Language Learning and Education, 9*(1), 14–20.

Index